MW00880483

Methods to Meals: Protein First Recipes You Will Love

supporting your **weight loss** surgery **health** management **goals** one **delicious** meal at a time

By *Kaye Bailey*

Kaye Bailey

On the front cover clockwise from top right: You Have Arrived Chicken and Shrimp, page 121; Wings to Fly For, page 94; Turkey and Eggs Chilled Lunch Plate, page 146; Kaye's Chicken Parmesan, page 91; Lemony Chicken Soup, page 69; Holiday Prime Rib Roast of Beef, page 156.

Cooking with Kaye

Methods to Meals: Protein First Recipes You Will Love

*supporting your weight loss surgery
health management goals
one delicious meal at a time*

Health Advice: The health content in *Cooking with Kaye* is intended to inform, not prescribe, and is not meant to be a substitute for the advice and care of a qualified health-care professional. The author and publisher disclaim any liability arising directly or indirectly from the use of this book.

Nutritional Analysis: Every effort has been made to check the accuracy of the nutritional information that appears with each recipe. However, because numerous variables account for a wide range of values for certain foods, nutritive analyses in this book should be considered approximate. Different results may be obtained by using different nutrient databases and different brand-name products.

This LivingAfterWLS publication November 2012; January 2017.

Proudly written, produced and manufactured in the United States of America.
LivingAfterWLS, LLC
Post Office Box 311
Evanston, WY 82931

Printed by CreateSpace, An Amazon.com Company

ISBN-13: 978-1542363730

A LivingAfterWLS Publication

Table of Contents

Important Note: Serving Size

For purposes of continuity recipe serving size and nutrient values are calculated and measured on the Daily Values standard for a 2,000 calorie/day diet for adults, developed by the Food and Drug Administration (FDA). It is understood that people who have undergone a restrictive bariatric surgical procedure will eat less than the standard serving size, and that people with different bariatric procedures will eat different volumes of food per serving. Please use the serving size and nutrient values provided as the baseline factor from which to calculate and adjust your specific and unique dietary intake.

Featured Articles Index

Introduction and Appreciation:

Thank you for joining me in the kitchen. This cookbook has been 13 years in the making and the result you now hold is the distillation of my own kitchen experiments *–many disasters and successes–* and endless research. Indeed, this work comes from the joyful pursuit of finding a cooking style that is suited to a blended household where people with their original organic tummies break bread at the table they share with one of us dining on our bariatric hybrid tummy.

For the last decade I have worked in the weight loss surgery community as a mentor encouraging and empowering my fellow patients to harness their inner strength and use the WLS tool as a means to healthy weight management and improved health and wellness. This work has fueled the fire within me to pursue excellence in the kitchen where I worked to develop the skills necessary to follow the WLS high protein, low carbohydrate eating plan in a manner that harmonizes the needs of our gastric-blended household.

The Process

I was not a good cook before surgery and I seldom followed a recipe. Our usual evening meal featured overcooked meat with potatoes or noodles smothered in condensed soup gravy. Sometimes I'd fancy things up a bit and microwave frozen vegetables, a disappointing attempt at bringing color to the plate. When I underwent gastric bypass surgery in 1999 I promised my husband that he *and* our misfit collection of frequent dinner guests *--kids and grandkids; neighbors, friends, and the random shirttail relatives arriving in bombastic fashion like traveling gypsies–* I promised him that we would continue to eat well and eat abundantly: the surgery wasn't going to change that. Perhaps you made a similar promise? My promise, however, was not without caveat: the surgery would be the catalyst for me to usher our meals in a new direction. I embarked on an intensive self-guided study program believing knowledge would empower me to make informed nutritional choices. We would focus on the quality of the food rather than quantity. I dedicated time to planning, preparing, and presenting meals and I enjoyed every minute of it.

The very nature of cooking is repetition; there are no original one-of a kind creations on the dinner plate. You and I, chopping and stirring and cooking in our kitchens: we are the accumulation of all the cooks who came before us since the beginning of time. Each generation takes from the past and gives to the future and thus tradition is born. I am thankful for countless cooks, professional chefs, authors, and mentors who guided me down the path to becoming a skilled and enthusiastic home cook.

I know with certainty that all of us will occasionally feel excluded from the traditions we treasure because our bariatric procedure has changed everything for us while the world around us stayed the same. I know this because sometimes I still feel left out of the good times I once celebrated with gusto. I know with equal conviction that with awareness and effort we can join that world from which we feel excluded, participating fully, *but differently,* from how we participated prior to our medical procedure. Within this book you will find ways to accommodate and nurture your sometimes misunderstood WLS peculiarities while fully participating in this great tradition we call living.

Appreciation

Perhaps it is silly, but I credit television instructional cooking shows for teaching me many kitchen skills. I am grateful for Martha Stewart who followed Julia Child in elevating the skills and knowledge of the home cook. Other TV instructors deserving thanks are Tyler Florence, Ellie Krieger, Bobby Flay, Sara Moulton, and Jacques Pépin.

As much as I enjoyed the beauty of visual learning from food television, the heart and soul of my inner scholar belongs to books. My grandmother started my cookbook collection in 1986 giving me The New Betty Crocker Cookbook. Today I enjoy more than 160 food spattered dog-eared volumes. Beginning with basic how-to instruction manuals, then advancing to food science textbooks and gourmet recipe collections, finally ending in a blast of glorious food photography masterpieces: I love them all.

In appreciation I mention a few favorite authors who made life-changing contributions to my culinary skill set with their teaching and sharing: Betsy Oppenner (Celebration Breads); Shirley O. Corriher (Cookwise: The Hows and Whys of Successful Cooking); Madeleine Kamman (The Making of a Cook); Denise Austin, fitness and healthy lifestyle coach; Molly Stevens (All About Braising); Mireille Guiliano, (French Women Don't Get Fat); Jamie Purviance (Weber grilling books); Bobby Flay (Food Network Chef and Bar Americain); Art Smith (Back to the Table); Dr. David Katz (The Way to Eat); Barbara Kafka,(Roasting and Soup: A Way of Life). This is but a short list of the influential teachers –*cooks and authors*- in my ongoing quest for culinary excellence in the home kitchen. I have included an extensive bibliography in the end pages and hope you will find some of these sources as beneficial as I have.

In the company of these inspiring cooks and chefs is the person who inspires me daily, my husband Jim. He drove me 1,500 miles away from home for this surgery and he has never left my side since. In the spirit of adventure and honoring his creed that life is for living he brings joy to our table and a hungry appetite for taste testing my latest culinary experiment. When you enjoy the recipes found here you can be certain they were improved upon at some point by suggestions from Jim. My extended time of learning and experimentation would not have been possible with anyone else. He has been a remarkably good sport about my culinary experiments never complaining when the clock strikes 10, my recipe has gone rogue, and the only thing I have to serve is a stale piece of cheese and short pour of old vine red. My husband loved me when I was a big girl and he loves me still today. I appreciate and adore this man who taught me by example that life is for living. And so I am, living in love, *and* LivingAfterWLS.

Thank you for joining me in *Methods to Meals*. I cannot wait to see what we can create together.

CHEERS!

Kaye
KayeBailey@LivingAfterWLS.com

Please Share: Pinterest

 In the spirit of connection and collaboration I invite you to share stories and pictures of the things you create that were inspired by *Methods to Meals*. We have a dedicated board on Pinterest: let's connect and cultivate a new tradition of sharing our experiences gleaned from *Methods to Meals*. See you there!

http://pinterest.com/kayebaileylawls

Whatever else you have on your mind,

Wherever else you think you are going,

Stop for a moment,

Look Where You Are:

You Have Arrived

LivingAfterWLS Creed

Mastering
Methods *to*
Meals

<blockquote>
"Recipes are like folktales, small parcels of culture. The history of cooking in many ways is like the history of language or the history of folk music - *a matter of borrowing, adapting, evolving.* The passing of a recipe is as important to cooking as the passing on of an idiom is important to the language."

Martha Stewart
</blockquote>

Mastering Methods to Meals

I have been eager to compile *Cooking with Kaye: Methods to Meals* for several years, inspired by the favorable feedback I receive from readers of our email newsletter *Cooking with Kaye*. The cooking newsletter, along with the other LivingAfterWLS ezine publications, magnified the borderless nature of our community where strangers with nothing else in common understand one another in a profoundly personal way. We are all trying to lose excess weight and manage our health in the exact same environment in which we became obese. Without exception, we share the fundamental desire to use bariatric surgery for weight management and we want to feel normal and stay sane in this crazy world where it is much easier to be fat.

It seems ironic that our basic need for nutrition, the very fuel that sustains all activities of life and living, is the thing we are least likely to give thought, time, and attention. Imagine what we can accomplish when higher priority is assigned to the preparation and enjoyment of nurturing meals.

Diversity: for all that we have in common we are also radically diverse. Our global community includes professional chefs and nutritionists; working moms and dads and babysitting grandparents: we have single people, old people, young people, sane people and few whack-a-doodles too. By virtue of one common denominator we connect with fry cooks, school teachers, dog walkers and World Wide Web food bloggers: novice home cooks, food lovers, and the culinary disinterested. We are sick and dying: we are healthy and living. I know diabetics, heart patients, disease fighters and disease survivors. They mingle with yoga masters, power lifters, the ladies from Curves® and marathon runners. We have picky eaters and carnivores; organic vegans and egg-eating vegetarians. We enjoy the free spirited "make-my-own-rules-selectarians" [sic] who tend to cluster with the sentimental crowd that has taken a stand against eating anything that lived *(or died)* wearing eyelashes or fur. Diversity indeed.

Our population is propelled to collect information from all manner of resources, internalize and digest it, and then map a path forward empowered by knowledge. I witness this daily in WLS pre-ops, post-ops, newbies, and veterans. In fact, you probably connected with me or a LivingAfterWLS Neighbor when you were seeking knowledge. As I set about planning this collection of method recipes I realized our diverse group will bring all manner of culinary skills when they join me in the kitchen, book in hand, ready to make a meal. To that conclusion, I have made every effort to write concise and thorough directions in order that both the novice and the skilled cook achieve equally successful results. I crafted this work as a tool for the many speaking with the voice and heart of one. I hope it serves you well as a text and tool: equal parts culinary science, liberal arts, and personal passion.

Before surgery my culinary joy came from eating. After surgery, my joy is in the art and science of composing a meal knowing it will provide sustenance to those who partake. If you believe what you read in popular media most people are put upon to prepare a meal and consider kitchen work an inconvenient disruption: drudgery of the lowliest kind. The popular antidote to such suffering shaves time off the task so the duration of unpleasant toil only hurts for a minute. Mainstream media is selling speed cooking besting the popular 30 minute meal with the 20 minute meal. And not long ago I saw the 10 minute meal is getting headline coverage promising to get us in and out of the kitchen faster than you can update your social media status.

It seems ironic that our basic need for nutrition, the very fuel that sustains all activities of life and living, is the thing we are least likely to give thought, time, and attention. In our task-driven days the one thing we sacrifice is properly fueling the engine that runs the body. Imagine what we can accomplish when higher priority is assigned to the preparation and enjoyment of nurturing meals.

Another thing ruffles me about instant meals and speed cooking: when we prepare a meal at frantic pace we tend to eat the meal at the same pace. One national food producer sells convenience products barking the slogan *"Get in: Get out; Get on with your life."* Has it really come to this? A more reasonable approach for me is *"Get in: Have Purpose; Nurture your life."*

In **Back to the Table** Art Smith, former personal chef to Oprah Winfrey, writes, "Dining together allows us to better understand who we are. [It] allows us to love and nurture each other and renew connections to our families – however they may be configured in this diverse and ever-changing society. One of the best ways I know to restore that daily balance is to sit down at the table. The table is a familiar, uncomplicated, and friendly place where we can celebrate family, friends, food, and life's many blessings." (Smith, 2001) I embrace this point of view in my life, and share it with you in **Methods to Meals.**

I have tested each recipe at least three times working in my unremarkable home kitchen. Testing recipes serves double duty for me: it is part of my job and we get to eat my work. To that end, like so many others, I prepare our evening meal while listening to the evening news, answering the phone, searching for lost kitchen tools; connecting, texting, and; bumbling about and losing my place in the recipe; cleaning up broken eggs. I test recipes in this insanely real environment because I know you will be preparing your meals in your own style of daily chaos. The following are hints for using **Methods to Meals**:

Pace of Preparation:

In holding true to my belief that meals are more than an inconvenient disruption I've taken away the usual stop-watch timetables for preparation and cooking. I don't like to race the clock and I find that when I do the meal falls short of enjoyable. The clock continues to tick despite the variables we cannot control. In **Methods to Meals** I have assigned the recipes one of three grades I call the "Pace of Preparation," a ballpark estimate of time from start to serving. I understand that, yes, we do need to prepare meals quickly much of the time. But I also understand that quick meals can meet our nutritional and budgetary needs and be delicious and satisfying as well.

> Each recipe is identified by Pace of Preparation just below the title line.

The Pace of Preparation is a travel metaphor. As we travel the highways and byways getting from here to there we know there are different routes to the same destination. Each route offers unique attributes and drawbacks. A Sunday drive can be refreshing, but not when we have a dozen errands to complete with no time to spare. And freeway scenery is rarely picturesque, but many times we must take the most efficient route to get from here to there

↦ **Indy Chef**   ⇄ **Freeway Chef**   ☼ **Country Road Chef**

The same goes for our meals. The destination is always the same: a thoughtfully prepared nutritious meal. The routes are different. Just like mapping a road trip with a destination the goal, we can plan the route to dinner based on the time available and needs of the day. Consider the three grades of Pace of Preparation:

⮂ Indy Chef:

Indy Chef meals are quick fix recipes that take advantage of ready-to-eat products, no-cook ingredients, and simple preparation techniques with minimal clean-up required. But don't let the speed fool you: ⮂ Indy Chef recipes are nutritionally balanced to sustain alertness and energy on busy nights when nothing else will do.

⇄ Freeway Chef:

Like the swift-moving divided highway, Freeway Chef recipes are an efficient way to get from preparation to meal without relentless starts, stops, and side trips. Use these recipes for their efficiency in preparation: enjoy them for their hunger-taming deliciousness and nutritional power. Most of the recipes in *Methods to Meals* are graded ⇄ Freeway Chef.

✿ Country Road Chef:

As much about the journey as the destination, Country Road Chef recipes are those slow leisurely meals holidays and Sundays are made of. Think family gatherings, special occasions, and just-because Sundays. Like a meandering drive down a country road these meals slow down the pace giving us time to enjoy the view. Take a break from the work-a-day and enjoy an occasional ✿Country Road Chef meal.

Please note: The Pace of Preparation refers to the overall timeframe in which a meal is prepared. When certain recipe steps must be timed precisely for the meal to be prepared successfully the timing is stated in the directions. For best results, please follow the directions closely.

Snapshots, Sidebars, Hints

Just below the recipe title line, aligned to the right, is the *Snapshot:* a quick look at the recipe attributes. You will find the icon for Pace of Preparation, and short descriptive phrases about the recipe. *Sidebars:* when appropriate recipe sidebars feature key learning points about ingredients, methods, nutrition, and our weight loss surgery lifestyle. Use these to build your knowledge base and expand your approach to meal planning and food preparation. Additional hints are offered following the directions: These suggestions are intended to inspire variations on the recipe and make good use of leftovers.

In most of my recipes you will not find salt and pepper on the ingredient list but the directions may instruct "season with salt and pepper." Baking aside, I have yet to meet someone who actually measures salt or pepper in cooking. Some cookbooks instruct us "season to taste" which seems redundant: if I am instructed to season with salt and pepper I will add salt and pepper to my liking, *to my taste*. Enjoy the freedom and make the recipe to your liking. Please note, if salt or pepper is a listed ingredient it should be measured and included as directed because it is necessary for a chemical process in the cooking.

We know that a diet high in sodium contributes to heart disease, stroke, and premature death. The Dietary Guidelines for Americans created by the U.S. Department of Agriculture adjusted the recommended daily intake of sodium in 2011 lowering it to 2300mg /day for adults. Lowering salt intake improves our cardiovascular health and reduces the risk of heart attack and stroke. One teaspoon of table salt is equivalent to 2300mg. Most of our dietary salt intake comes from canned and processed foods. I use reduced sodium products whenever possible in hopes of reducing our hidden sodium intake. Use the products that are suited to your sodium requirements. When canned beans are used the instructions state to rinse and drain: this washes some of the sodium away before including them in the meal.

Cooking Spray

You will notice I do not list cooking spray in the ingredient list of the recipes, but the directions may call for using cooking spray in the method. It is assumed most home cooks keep cooking spray on hand and use it following label directions. When the recipe directions specify a flavored cooking spray such as butter flavor or olive oil flavor it is because the added flavor enhances the dish. This is the cook's choice and flavorless cooking spray works for all preparations.

Sugar, Honey, and Everything Sweet

I think we are all anxious about sugar after bariatric surgery, and with good cause considering the potential this simple ingredient has to disrupt our best weight management effort. It no longer surprises me to receive emails from concerned readers questioning a recipe that includes sugar or honey. A sweetener such as sugar, brown sugar, honey, jam, jelly, or preserves is called for when it is needed to affect a chemical reaction that will enhance the flavors and textures of other ingredients. A small amount of sugar added to protein facilitates browning and searing to bring out the rich succulent flavor of the meat. Tomato sauce based recipes often call for sugar which balances the acidity to produce a smoother sauce. The grams of sugar per serving are generally reported as "trace amounts" and are unlikely to impact blood glucose levels.

If you absolutely must omit the sweetener called for do not substitute artificial sweetener. Artificial sweeteners do not share the same reactive properties with sugar. When heat is introduced they tend to taint food with a bitter metallic taste.

And there may be more cause for concern about artificial sweeteners. In early 2012 the diabetes and weight loss experts at the Mayo Clinic issued a warning to diabetics advising some products labeled as diet, diabetic or sugar-free contain sweeteners with calories and carbohydrates that may affect one's blood sugar level. They also shared evidence that products made with artificial low-calorie sweeteners may lead to increased calorie intake and weight gain.

Label Reading Memory Trick: Food labels report added sugar in grams, but in our kitchens we measure sugar by volume in measuring spoons or by the cup. A simple conversion to remember when looking at labels is 4 to 1: four grams of sugar to 1 teaspoon of sugar. Just like 4 quarters make 1 dollar.

Optional, To Taste, If Desired

In developing and writing recipes and then sharing them with you I am telling you *"This is how I make this dish for our table."* When I share a recipe I expect the cook who replicates it will make it as they see fit. It amuses me to read recipes that grant permission by instructing, "Garnish with parsley, *if desired.*" I can honestly say I like parsley and I appreciate it as a pretty garnish. But I do not desire, long for, wish for, or even yearn for parsley; my apologies to the humble herb but I just don't have those kind of feelings. When following my recipes please take all the liberties you desire and deem appropriate: adjust to taste. If you don't have an ingredient or if you don't care for an ingredient adjust, omit, substitute. You are perfectly free to do anything you wish in the privacy of your own kitchen, if you so *desire.*

Vinaigrettes and Marinades: Do use care when adjusting ingredients in vinaigrettes and marinades. Recipes that contain oil and vinegar must maintain the correct ratio of acid and oil in order for the ingredients to properly emulsify.

Alcohol: Recipes that call for alcohol need the liquid to tenderize protein or impart rich flavor to the recipe. If you elect to cook without alcohol the correct substitution for beer is an equal measure apple cider (not apple juice). To replace wine in recipes use broth suited to the other ingredients and consider adding 1 to 2 teaspoons of red wine vinegar or white wine vinegar to replace red or white wine, respectively.

Weights and Measures

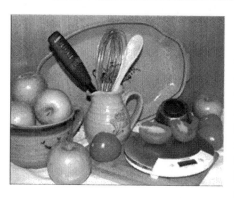

A few simple tools for weights and measures are essential to a carefully managed diet. My tools are workhorses and I work them hard. If we want to ensure the accuracy of our recipe we need to measure the ingredients instead of guessing or free pouring. Studies show that cooks who free pour oil into the skillet add 65 percent more calories to the recipe than cooks who measure according to recipe directions. Equip your kitchen with measuring spoons and measuring cups. Keep them in a convenient spot where you instinctively reach for them before you pour.

Weighted measure is also important because most of our protein intake is measured by weight. I use a battery operated digital scale *(shown above measuring the weight of a sliced tomato)*. To ensure cleanliness I keep a handy box of single-sheet deli wax paper near the scale. Placing this nearly weightless barrier between the scale and the ingredient is an efficient method for protecting surfaces from contamination. A quality kitchen scale runs about $25 and can be found in department stores, big retailers, and bath and kitchen stores.

Meat Thermometer: I am a big believer in getting the meat cooked correctly so it is appealing to eat and not lost to the waste of improper cooking. The best way I know to guarantee perfectly cooked meat is using a quality meat thermometer. I use an instant-read digital thermometer made by Weber (shown above in the utensil caddy): it is priced under $20. The thermometer has a long probe which is inserted to the center of the meat and a digital display promptly reveals the internal temperature in Fahrenheit or Celsius. Refer to the Internal Cooking Temperatures chart on page 181 for the U.S.

Department of Agriculture safe cooking guidelines. A meat thermometer is a small investment that nets big rewards!

Stay Sharp

There is nothing more frustrating to me in the kitchen than a dull knife. Dull knives are inefficient and they are more dangerous than sharp knives because they must be manipulated with force to accomplish the task of

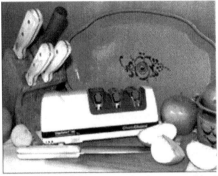

cutting or chopping. Many people sharpen their knives with a stone or the sharpening steel that often comes with the set of knives. Jim is the knife-master in our home and he uses an electric knife sharpener by Chef's Choice *(shown above)*. While the initial investment of about $120-$200 (depending on model) seems steep, in the long run well-cared for properly sharpened knifes will last a lifetime.

After 16 years of use our knives wear the patina of age. The set was affordable: arrogant gourmets who spend hundreds of dollars on knives might even call them cheap. But because they are well maintained (hand washed, sharpened regularly, handles oiled) they make the task of chopping, slicing, mincing, and dicing efficient and safe. That is the very definition of a good knife.

It is not necessary to amass a collection of task-specific knives, according to Madeleine Kamman in "The New Making of a Cook." In fact, she declares there are only four knives essential to the well-equipped home kitchen (Kamman, 1997). They include:

- 9 to 10-inch chef's knife for chopping vegetables
- 2 to 3-inch blade paring knife for paring and boning.
- Bendable-blade fileting knife
- 12 to 14-inch blade slicing knife for carving cooked and uncooked meats

Cutting Boards: Knives should always be used on clean cutting boards dedicated to their purpose. Most cooks have one cutting board for vegetables and fruits and a second board for raw meats, fish, and poultry. Using dedicated cutting boards is a good safeguard against food borne illness caused by cross contamination. To keep cutting boards clean, the USDA recommends washing them with hot, sudsy water after each use; then rinse in hot running water and air-dry. I am currently using bamboo cutting boards: they are durable, lightweight, and air-dry quickly.

Speaking of sanitation, do you know that many weight loss surgery post-ops experience increased susceptibility to food illness after surgery? Experts are flummoxed to understand why our susceptibility increases but they are clear that vigilant kitchen hygiene will prevent food borne illness. Cleaning and sanitizing surfaces requires two steps to effectively kill germs and microorganisms. First, wash the surface with hot soapy water; rinse thoroughly with water. Next, apply a sanitizing solution to the surface. Allow the solution to sit for a few minutes before wiping clean with dry paper towels. Always follow label instructions.

It's Your Turn

I say this often: *We are all in this together.* Now it is your turn. Throughout the five method and recipe chapters you will discover pages with room to write your recipe. I hope you will include your culinary creations in this book and consider it a collaboration well done. Should the sharing mood strike I'd love to receive your recipe to add to my collection.

Email me: KayeBailey@LivingAfterWLS.com

The Four Rules of Weight Loss Surgery

Protein First

Lots of Water

NO SNACKING

daily

eXercise

Meat: beef, bison, lamb, game. The term meat is a broadly used term that includes beef, bison, lamb, and game meat. Beef is the most commonly consumed meat in the United States while lamb is the top in meat consumption worldwide. Bison or buffalo is becoming more readily available with the increase of agricultural bison ranches. Bison and game may be substituted for beef in most recipes. People following a high protein diet should select lean cuts of meat to reduce their intake of saturated fat.

Poultry. Chicken, turkey and other poultry are popular sources of lean protein for their ease in preparation and affordability. White meat poultry contains less fat than dark meat, but dark meat protein is a better source of nutrients including B vitamins.

Pork. There is much talk about today's leaner pork thanks to improved agriculture practices. Lean cuts such as tenderloin, top loin, rib chops, and sirloin steak are 31 percent leaner than the same cuts two decades ago. Pork cooks quickly and is affordably priced similar to chicken.

Fish and shellfish. Perhaps the best source of lean protein combined with healthy fats, fish and shellfish support a well-planned high protein diet. Most fish contain the heart-healthy fat known as omega 3 which is shown to improve cardiovascular health and prevent the risk of stroke and heart disease.

Soy. Plant based soy protein, the base ingredient for tofu, is a low-fat protein option with the added benefit of cholesterol lowering properties.

Beans and legumes. High protein diets tend to be low in dietary fiber. Including beans and legumes in meals provides the benefits of plant protein and dietary fiber in one healthy ingredient. A half cup serving of beans contains nearly the same protein as 3 ounces of broiled steak.

Low-fat dairy. Milk, cheese, and yogurt are not only protein-rich; they also provide calcium for strong bones and a healthy heart. Low-fat, or reduced fat dairy products provide the benefits of dairy with lowered calories.

Protein First:
A really big deal in our long-term WLS success

Prior to most bariatric procedures patients are taught Four Rules that we agree to follow for the rest of our life. The Four Rules[1] are misleading in their simplicity: Protein First; Lots of Water; No Snacking; Daily Exercise. Fewer than ten words! I remember being so overwhelmed by the transition that surgery puts in motion that I was grateful for the simplicity of these four little guidelines. But as time marched forward and weight loss became more difficult and later weight maintenance was confusing and illusive I became desperate for more information. I needed details so I could intelligently sustain a healthy weight and manage my WLS tool. Leaving my weight management to chance had never worked before surgery and I was fearful that after surgery leaving things to chance would take me right back up the scale to morbid obesity.

So, it turns out, *Protein First* is highly critical in our weight management efforts. Not just in the early days and weeks following surgery, but for as long as we live. And *Protein First* sounds simple and easy but we quickly

> A protein-rich diet can lead to increased satiety, enhanced weight loss, and improved body composition.

discover the information about protein can be confusing and complicated. Before we hit the pots and pans in the recipe section of this cookbook we need to review why Protein *First* is a really big deal in our long-term success. This knowledge works in concert with the recipes so you can manage your WLS tool and never have to surrender your weight management to chance.

A weight loss surgery *Protein First* diet is a high protein diet. This indicates that of the three major nutrients (protein, fat, and carbohydrate) protein contributes 50 percent or more of our food intake, followed by fat and carbohydrates in near-equal percentages. The National Academies of Sciences (NAS) defines the Recommended Dietary Allowance (RDA) for protein at 56 grams for men and 46 grams for women. Most nutritionists agree this recommendation is invalid because it is based on decades-old data when humans weighed less. This standard is set using the mid-20th century census when the average body weight for men was 156 pounds and women 126 pounds. We are heavier today: 2010 data reveals the median weight for men is 191 pounds, a 35 pound gain. The median weight for women is 164

---

[1] See Appendix A: WLS Four Rules and Basic Tenets on page 176.

pounds, a 38 pound increase. Since our protein needs are directly related to body weight most of us are outside the parameters set by NAS.

Adding to our confusion, bariatric nutritionists are not in agreement about post-op protein intake. In fact, a 2008 study reveals nutritionists recommend anywhere from 60 to 105 grams of protein a day for patients following a 1,200-calorie diet. (Swilley, 2008). These recommendations appear to be random and lack congruity regarding procedure, gender, initial weight, goal weight, BMI, age, or geographical region.

Vague and inconsistent information abounds. That coupled with the pouch discomfort or tightness associated with eating protein, makes this simple *Protein First* rule a real puzzler. Why, just give a shout-out to your online WLS support group asking *"How much protein should we be eating each day?"* and the replies you receive will include a plethora of specific numbers and a variety of creative mathematical formulas to calculate protein requirements. It's no wonder we become frustrated and often simply leave our nutrition to chance and hope for the best. But hoping for the best isn't working for many of us; we are not eating the amount of protein our bodies need for optimum health, weight loss, and weight maintenance. In fact, recent studies of bariatric post-ops confirm insufficient protein intake is putting our health at risk.

In 2011 a leading researcher and bariatric specialist reported, "We found that there have been few studies on protein intake recommendations for bariatric patients. Dietary protein ingestion among this population tends to be inadequate, potentially leading to a loss of lean body mass, reduced metabolic rates, and physiological damage. Conversely, a protein-rich diet can lead to increased satiety, enhanced weight loss, and improved body composition. The quality and composition of protein sources are also very important." (Silvia Leite Faria, Et.Al, 2011)

Daily Protein Intake (DPI)

Good news came later in 2011 when a large study confirmed that compliance with a set Daily Protein Intake (DPI) resulted in increased weight loss, decreased body fat, and an increased percentage of lean body mass. "Excellent compliance with a DPI of more than 1 gram protein for each kilogram of body weight is feasible and will likely result in the benefits of increased weight loss, a decreased percentage of body fat, and improved percentage of lean mass." (Ioannis Raftopoulos; et al., 2011).

22

More importantly, the research produced a solid formula by which to determine our individual DPI. We can now calculate our individual protein requirement with a formula based on science and proven with a credible four-year study of nearly 500 bariatric post-operative patients. The formula is straightforward: two simple calculations. Knowing our individual protein needs is a great starting point for ongoing successful weight management I've added a chart to make your record keeping a snap.

> In plain language, we need to eat at minimum of 1 gram of protein, preferably more, for every kilogram we weigh.

Daily Protein Intake it is simply a ratio of body weight in kilograms to protein intake in grams. In all cases after weight loss surgery our DPI should be ≥1g/kg/day. In plain language, every day we need to eat at least 1 gram of protein, preferably more, for every kilogram we weigh.

Personalize your DPI

First we must convert our weight in pounds to kilograms with this formula: (pounds ÷ 2.2 = kilograms). Next, using the table on page 25 we should identify our Protein Factor based on age or health condition. This is the formula for your personalized Daily Protein Intake:

(lbs. ÷ 2.2 = kg) (kg x Protein Factor = protein grams/day)

Let's look at a specific example. Shelly currently weighs 216 pounds after losing 80 pounds with the help of gastric bypass. She would like to continue to lose weight by following the Four Rules, especially *Protein First*. Here are her calculations using the upper end of the Protein Factor for weight loss:

(216 ÷ 2.2=98kg) (98 x 1.8 = 176 grams protein/day)

Shelly needs to eat 176 grams of protein a day! Shockingly, this body-specific formula nearly quadruples the RDA for women of 46 grams of protein per day set by the NAS. Based on current science we know that the standard RDA of 46 grams of protein will not nurture good health for Shelly, nor will it promote weight loss. Shelly will achieve much better results using her personalized DPI. On the front lines of nutrition these old guidelines are being discarded and we are seeing this patient-specific formula used by an increasing number of bariatric centers and mainstream nutritionists.

Some experts suggest creating a DPI range rather than a single specific number for daily intake. This makes sense. Who wouldn't be intimidated and discouraged by the very thought of eating 176 grams of protein a day? It seems like an impossible target to hit. It is far more encouraging to create a range in which our Daily Protein Intake should fall. A target range gives us some *Protein First* wiggle room that feels encouraging and achievable. Establishing a range is easy to do using two Protein Factors to calculate a high and low end. This is what Shelly's DPI window for weight loss looks like using Protein Factors 1.4 (low) and 1.8 (high):

Shelly's DPI for *weight loss* at 216 pounds:
137-176 grams protein/day
Low-end: (216 ÷ 2.2=98kg) (98 x 1.4 = 137g DPI)
High-end: (216 ÷ 2.2=98kg) (98 x 1.8 = 176g DPI)

With a 40-gram window to work with Shelly was able to meet her protein intake goals fairly consistently and she is now down to 160 pounds, the weight she would like to maintain. As she begins a lifelong pursuit of healthy weight management she will adjust her Daily Protein Intake. For weight maintenance she used Protein Factors 1.2 and 1.6 respectively. Here's how the numbers shake out:

Daily Protein Intake
≥1 g/kg/day

Pounds ÷ 2.2 = Kilograms
Kilograms x Protein Factor = DPI

Shelly's DPI for *weight maintenance* at 160 pounds: 86g-115g DPI
(160 ÷ 2.2=72kg) (72 x 1.2 = 86g DPI)
(160 ÷ 2.2=72kg) (72 x 1.6 = 115g DPI)

This formula is effective because we can adjust it as our weight changes or if we are not getting the desired results of weight loss or weight maintenance. During weight loss I suggest a review and recalculation with every 10-pound change in body weight. You are the manager of your DPI range. If you set your DPI window and consistently consume an amount of protein within that range, but do not get the results you want then take another look and adjust the numbers. The experts know that we each have our own DPI for weight loss and we can find it using this proven formula. It is up to us to find that personal magic number.

It is based on research findings that nutritionists developed the Protein Factor. While the governing agencies including the FDA, CDC, and NAS have been slow to adopt the Protein Factor, many nutritionists are using it with pleasing results. The Protein Factor is selected based on age, level of activity, or current health condition:

Protein Factor Daily Protein Intake	
Age or Condition	**Grams Protein Per Kilograms of Weight** [2]
Adults, 19 to 50 years old	0.9 to 1.2
Adults over 50	1.0 to 1.5
For weight loss	1.0 to 1.8
Recreational athletes	1.2 to 1.4
Endurance athletes	1.2 to 1.7
Strength training athletes	1.7 to 1.8
For rheumatoid arthritis [3]	1.5 to 2.0
For infections, fractures, fever, surgery [3]	2.0
For severe trauma, wound healing, burns [3]	2.5 – 3.0

Now let's discover how much protein you need each day.

A ÷ 2.2 = B
(Body Weight pounds)**A** ÷ 2.2 = Body Weight (kilograms) **B**

Refer to the table to find your condition. To calculate the maximum DPI select the higher number, in the case of Protein Factor for Weight Loss the number is 1.8. Multiply body weight in kilograms by the Protein Factor you selected, shown here as PF1:

B X PF1 = DPI
Body Weight (kilograms) **B** x Protein Factor **PF1** = _____ **Max. DPI/grams**

Next, select the Protein factor on the low side to find your minimum DPI. Again for weight loss we see the number is 1.0: this is PF2:

B X PF2 = DPI
Body Weight (kilograms) **B** x Protein Factor **PF2** = _____ **Min. DPI/grams**

---

[2] Recommendations based on normal kidney function. People suffering renal disease should follow the diet prescribed by their nephrologist or renal care team.

[3] When suffering these conditions please follow the specific guidelines and health management instructions provided by your doctor or nutritionist.

Enter your personal numbers and the date below. This is the benchmark so that you can make dietary adjustments intelligently based on facts and record keeping: this is a new day of progress toward your goal! And I told you it was easy (I don't like to do math either!). Use this formula and table to update your information as necessary to change your results.

(Remember, you can always download our many charts and forms for free, go to LivingAfterWLS.com and click Downloads)

Date:	Body Weight Pounds/Kilograms	PF1 / Min. DPI/g	PF2 / Max. DPI/g	DPI Range
(Shelly's Data) 01/01/2012	*216lbs. / 98kg*	*1.4 / 137g*	*1.8 / 176g*	*137 – 176g*

2B/1B

(2 Bites Protein to 1 Bite Carbohydrate)

Protein

salads FIRST

> You need four people to make a salad:
> One to add oil lavishly,
> One to add vinegar parsimoniously,
> One to add salt wisely,
> And a madman to toss it a thousand times
> And that's how you dress a salad.
> *Italian Proverb*

2B/1B *Protein First* Salads

Methods and Articles:

Recipes:

↦ **Indy Chef**   ⇆ **Freeway Chef**   ✿ **Country Road Chef**

So you want to eat salad after WLS? Here's how:

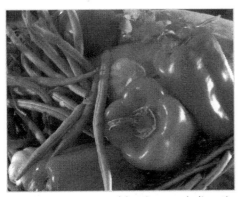

A trip to the salad bar after weight loss surgery sometimes feels more like a trek through a minefield than a healthy meal solution. Weight loss surgery procedures cause a decreased production of digestive enzymes: the result is a compromised ability to digest certain raw fruits and vegetables. Some people report extreme gas, bloating, and digestive discomfort after eating salad greens and other raw vegetables. For the first three years after my gastric bypass I could not eat any greens or raw vegetables because of the digestive upset they caused. Now, more than a decade later, there are days salad sits well and other days salad makes my pouch very grumpy. I know that many of my WLS Neighbors experience the same Moody Pouch Syndrome (MPS). From our collective experience I've learned if we compose our salads with a purposeful protein-fat-carbohydrate ratio we are more likely to enjoy them without suffering MPS.

If you will forgive my gender stereotype I would like to suggest we favor "Man Salads" forsaking the more feminine salad from our "lunching with ladies" pre-surgery days. Women build salads with a generous foundation of lettuce topped with petite bites of raw vegetables, a few grams of protein from boiled eggs or bacon bits, and we politely eat it with dressing on the side. Men, on the other hand, construct a salad with goodly amounts of protein: grilled steak or chicken for example. They pile-on cheese, bacon, eggs, shrimp, and salmon. They top this creation with a generous pour of dressing and garnish it with a leaf or two of lettuce. Picture a nicely made Cobb salad, easy on the lettuce, and you get the idea.

2B/1B Protein First Salads are built like the Man Salad. In conventional nutrition salads are composed of equal parts protein, fat, and carbohydrate. In bariatric nutrition the balance changes slightly: 2 parts protein to 1 part carbohydrate with healthy fats added sparingly. When we strive for a balance of two-thirds protein to one-third vegetables and fruit (complex carbohydrates) topped with a healthy dressing, we are likely to enjoy a meal that sits well in the pouch and meets our *Protein First* requirements.

These salad recipes are created to serve our unique WLS digestive system. After surgery we have a lower level of digestive enzymes which contributes to occasional discomfort and poor digestion when we eat salad and raw vegetables. In our WLS vernacular the expression 2B/1B Rhythm means we eat two bites of protein to one bite carbohydrate. Years ago I started the practice of counting bites, not grams or calories, because it is easy to do in most situations. When we follow the 2B/1B Rhythm we are eating *Protein First*. I call these 2B/1B *Protein First* Salads because the counting is built into the recipe. The ratio of 2-parts protein to 1-part carbohydrate translates to a 2B/1B rhythm. Feel free to count bites just to be sure.

> Count Bites:
> 2B/1B Rhythm
>
> 2 Bites Protein +
> 1 Bite Carbohydrate=
> Protein First Salad

Tips for creating 2B/1B Protein First Salads

Ready-to-Eat salad greens: In the last two decades grocers have transitioned from providing a large assortment of loose lettuce and salad greens to having only a few loose greens making room for convenient bagged salads. Packaging for freshness and sanitation is sophisticated and food regulatory agencies say salads labeled "washed", "triple washed" or "ready-to-eat" do not need additional washing at home (California Department of Public Health, 2010).

Because bagged greens are more common than loose lettuce I use cups for the unit of measure in these salad recipes instead of the more traditional measuring units of "head of lettuce" or "bunch of spinach." Look at the ingredient list on packaged salad and try to come close to the amount called for in the recipe. Bunched salad greens (not package salads) should also be measured by the cup. Knowing we have different tolerance levels for salad greens means we should adjust the measurement to suit our needs.

All Dressed Up: Do **not** use fat free dressings; they do not contribute any nutrition. Studies show that healthy monounsaturated fat, such as olive oil, is necessary for the absorption of vitamins and minerals. To promote the absorption of nutrients from the protein and carbohydrates include olive oil or other monounsaturated fat in your meal. Reduced calorie or reduced fat dressings are acceptable provided they are made with some healthy fat. You can't beat vinaigrettes when looking for a healthy salad dressing. Olive oil and balsamic vinegar, the primary ingredients in vinaigrettes, are known to support good health, aid nutrient absorption, and improve digestion.

Dietary Fats: Brief Review	
Studies support the prevailing nutritional belief that some varieties of fat, used sparingly, are beneficial to our health.	
Include these:	**Limit these:**
Monounsaturates found in olive, canola and peanut oils as well as most nuts and avocados.	**Saturated fats** are found in animal-based foods, such as meats, poultry, lard, egg yolks and whole-fat dairy products including butter and cheese. They're also in cocoa butter and coconut, palm and other tropical oils, which are used in many coffee lighteners, snack crackers, baked goods and other processed food.
Polyunsaturated fats are found in other plant-based oils, such as safflower, corn, sunflower, soybean, sesame and cottonseed oils.	**Trans-fats** also called partially hydrogenated vegetable oil – are found in hardened vegetable fats, such as stick margarine and vegetable shortening, and in foods made with them.

Dietary fat is used efficiently by the body as fuel. It is interesting to observe that fat intake is self-regulating and our bodies have a built-in "off" switch for fat consumption. "Few people would sit and eat a stick of butter, or swig olive oil by the cup," says Dr. Michael R. Eades who specializes in bariatric and weight loss medicine. He adds, "Without carbohydrates to wrap the fat around, eating fat not very appealing." (Michael R. Eades, 1996)

People who have drastically lowered or eliminated fat from their diet complain of constant nagging hunger. They are not imagining this hunger. Fat consumed with abundant protein and complex carbohydrates slows the stomach from emptying: we feel full longer. Lingering feelings of satiation prevent post-meal snacking and stomach rumbling. Salads dressed with flavorful vinaigrettes composed of healthy oil and beneficial vinegars support our healthy WLS diet.

Roast Beef and Blue Cheese Salad

☞ **Indy Chef, 5 ingredients, no cooking required, portable**

Enjoy the refreshing flavor and crunch of green salad while getting your *Protein First* in this easy-to-prepare plated salad. The ratio of greens to meat and cheese readily provides a generous serving that makes the 2B/1B count easily obtainable.

Ingredients:

8 cups salad greens, washed, ready-to-eat

16 ounces thinly sliced deli roast beef

1 pint cherry or grape tomatoes,

¼ cup (1-ounce) crumbled blue cheese

½ cup reduced calorie raspberry vinaigrette

Directions: For each serving arrange 2 cups of mixed greens on a dinner or salad plate. Divide roast beef into 4 stacks, 4-ounces each; roll jellyroll fashion and cut crosswise into 1-inch slices. Keep rolled and arrange the rolls from one 4-ounce stack atop the greens on each salad plate. Divide the tomatoes and blue cheese evenly among the four servings. Dress each salad with 1-2 tablespoons of the raspberry vinaigrette. Serve immediately.

> Lean beef is an excellent source of protein averaging 10 grams per ounce. In addition, one 3-ounce serving of beef provides goodly amounts of B vitamins, iron, and zinc. Each ounce of lean beef averages 61 calories.

Nutrition: 4 servings. Each serving provides 353 calories, 35 grams protein, 12 grams fat, 13 grams carbohydrate and 2 grams dietary fiber.

Try This: In place of deli roast beef use thinly sliced left-over roast beef or steak ~ Sprinkle 1 tablespoon toasted walnuts on each salad. ~ When transporting salad store the vinaigrette separately and dress salad just before serving. ~ Fresh raspberries or other seasonal berries are a healthy addition to this salad. Gently wash fresh raspberries, blackberries, blueberries or strawberries, pat dry, add ¼ cup to each salad just before dressing. ~ Toss fresh raspberries with vinaigrette; garnish salad with raspberries and dress with vinaigrette.

Grilled Beef, Red Onion and Blue Cheese Salad

⇆ Freeway Chef, grilled casual supper, company friendly, seasonal ingredients

The easy-to-make vinaigrette in this recipe plays double duty seasoning the steak before grilling and dressing the salad for serving. Use a screw-top jar and shake the vinaigrette ingredients into a delicious emulsified dressing.

Ingredients:

3 tablespoons balsamic vinegar

2 tablespoons olive oil

½ teaspoon minced bottled garlic or 1 clove garlic minced

1 (16-ounce) boneless beef top sirloin steak, cut 1-inch thick

1 tablespoon snipped fresh thyme

2 teaspoons snipped fresh rosemary

1 red onion, sliced into ¼-inch rings

6 cups salad greens, washed, ready-to-eat

1 pint cherry or grape tomatoes

¼ cup crumbled blue cheese

Food safety standards instruct beef should be cooked to a minimum internal temperature of 145°F to prevent food borne illness. Test cooked protein with instant-read digital thermometer for proper doneness. See page 181 for Safe Minimum Cooking Temperatures.

Directions: For vinaigrette, in a screw-top jar combine balsamic vinegar, oil, and garlic. Cover and shake well; season with salt and pepper. Trim fat from steak. Brush steak with 1 tablespoon of vinaigrette, press thyme and rosemary on steak. Set aside. Brush onion slices with vinaigrette; reserve remaining vinaigrette. Prepare grill to medium high heat. Grill steak to desired doneness over medium high heat keeping grill uncovered. Grill onion slices until tender and browned. Divide salad greens among 4 plates. Thinly slice steak across the grain and arrange on greens with grilled onion slices. Dress with vinaigrette and top with tomatoes and blue cheese

Nutrition: 4 servings. Each serving provides 266 calories, 28 grams protein, 16 grams fat, 9 grams carbohydrate and 2 grams dietary fiber.

Try This: Grill sliced fresh seasonal vegetables brushing with vinaigrette and serve with salad. ~ Use a variety of heirloom tomatoes in place of the cherry or grape tomatoes. ~ Save time: use prepared quality vinaigrette.

Southwestern Steak Salad

Bring the flavors of the southwest to your table with this casual dinner salad in which the grilled steak is the star. Rich in iron and protein, steak is a welcome addition to the *Protein First* meal.

Ingredients:

1 (16-ounce) beef top sirloin steak cut 1-inch thick, trimmed of fat

6 cups spinach greens, ready-to-eat

1 medium sweet red pepper, diced

1 (15-ounce) can black beans, rinsed and drained

1 medium ripe tomato, diced

1 bunch green onions, chopped

1 medium avocado, diced

½ cup ranch salad dressing, reduced calorie

½ cup salsa

1 teaspoon taco seasoning, low or no sodium

> Never underestimate the power of ready-to-eat commercial salsa. A spoonful added to dressing, gravy, soup or sauce takes bland to bold with very little effort. Go for it! Boring tasteless food is the demise of any well-intended meal.

Directions: Season steak with salt and pepper. On preheated grill cook steak over medium heat for 8-10 minutes per side or until meat reaches desired doneness. Remove steak from heat and allow to rest 5 minutes before carving. While steak cooks in a large bowl toss together the spinach, diced red pepper, black beans, diced tomato, chopped green onions, and diced avocado. In a small bowl whisk the ranch salad dressing with the salsa and taco seasoning. Carve the steak against the grain and serve with tossed salad and salsa-ranch dressing.

Nutrition: Serves 4. Each serving provides 517 calories, 29 grams protein, 33 grams fat, 27 grams carbohydrate, 10 grams dietary fiber.

Try This: Use grilled fish or poultry in place of the beef for a change of protein. ~ Brown ground beef seasoned with salt, pepper and taco seasoning for a taco salad variation. Arrange a salad bar with all ingredients and encourage everyone to compose their own salad.

Chicken and Chickpea Salad

🏳 Indy Chef, Mediterranean
flavors, convenient ingredients

The balance of fresh herbs and vegetables with the chicken makes this an ideal 2B/1B Salad. The salad may be prepared in advance and served plated, tucked in a pita, or rolled in a wrap. Chickpeas, sometimes called garbanzo beans, are a good source of vegetable protein and soluble fiber.

Ingredients:

1 (9-ounce) package cooked chicken breast, thawed, chopped or sliced

1 (15-ounce) can chickpeas, rinsed and drained

1 small cucumber, seeded and chopped

4 green onions, white parts only, chopped

¼ cup fresh mint or basil, chopped

½ cup plain fat-free yogurt

2 cloves garlic, minced

¼ teaspoon salt

2 cups spinach leaves, ready-to-eat

1/3 cup feta cheese, crumbled

1 lemon, cut into wedges

> Turn leftovers into tomorrow's tasty lunch by stuffing a whole grain or low-carb tortilla-type wrap with this salad. Refrigerate until serving and enjoy a fun *Protein First* brown bag meal.

Directions: In a large mixing bowl gently toss together the chicken, chickpeas, cucumber, green onions, mint (or basil), yogurt, garlic, and salt. If preparing to serve later cover and refrigerate at this point. Just before serving fold-in spinach leaves and crumbled feta cheese. Serve on chilled salad plates garnished with lemon wedges.

Nutrition: 4 servings. Each 1¾ cup serving provides 258 calories, 28 grams protein, 6 grams fat, 22 grams carbohydrate and 6 grams dietary fiber.

Try This: Use salad to fill a low-carb whole grain wrap or pita pocket for a convenient hand-held meal. ~ Try including a cup of red grapes, halved, in the salad mixture for a sweet flavor. ~ Use leftover roast turkey or chicken in place of the packaged cooked chicken breast.

Chopped Chicken Salad with Apples and Walnuts

⇆ Freeway Chef, big flavor,
convenient ingredients, easy assembly

This chicken salad has it all: crisp lettuce, sweet-tart apple, succulent chicken chunks, fresh vegetables, and crunchy walnuts. It rivals the best steak house main-course salad yet is simple enough to prepare and serve for a weeknight meal in a snap.

Ingredients:

8 cups mixed salad greens, ready-to-eat

2 cups cooked chicken, deboned and skinned, cut 1-inch cubes

1 (15-ounce) can great northern beans, rinsed and drained

2 tart apples, washed, cored and diced

1 medium cucumber, peeled and chopped

1 medium tomato, chopped

1 medium avocado, diced

2 ribs celery, sliced ¼-inch thick

1 bunch green onions, chopped

¼ cup chopped walnuts

bottled raspberry vinaigrette, reduced calorie

It is less expensive to prepare vinaigrette from scratch using pantry ingredients, but there are times convenience trumps cost and a bottled vinaigrette best meets our needs. Both homemade and well-made store dressings play a supporting role in our effort to keep flavors fresh and varied.

Directions: Arrange salad greens on large serving plate. In a large bowl gently toss together the chicken, great northern beans, apples, cucumber, tomato, avocado, celery and green onions. Arrange atop the salad greens. Sprinkle with chopped walnuts. Serve with vinaigrette on the side, dress salads following portion information on bottle.

Nutrition: Serves 4. Each serving provides 340 calories, 34 grams protein, 7 grams fat, 39 grams carbohydrate, 10 grams dietary fiber.

Kaye's Choice - Bottled Vinaigrette: When using commercially bottled vinaigrette I prefer Ken's Steak House Lite Raspberry Walnut Vinaigrette. Look for prepared vinaigrette with fewer than 100 calories per 2 tablespoon serving. Check for added sugars and know your personal tolerance or the sugar limit advised by your bariatric team. Define your personal nutrition needs and find products that meet those criteria.

Greek Chicken Salad with Feta and Olives

The Mediterranean flavors of this Greek-style salad take an average chicken salad beyond ordinary to exceptional. Using ready-to-eat ingredients from the market this salad is quick to prepare and beautiful to present.

Ingredients:

1 (12-ounce) package romaine lettuce, chopped, ready-to-eat

2 (6-ounce) packages refrigerated grilled chicken breast strips, chopped

2 pints grape tomatoes, halved

1 small cucumber, peeled, seeded, diced

1/3 cup reduced-fat feta cheese

1 (4.25-ounce) can sliced olives

½ medium red onion, thinly sliced

¼ cup reduced calorie olive oil vinaigrette

juice of ½ lemon; cut remaining half in wedges for garnish

This is a beautiful salad when it is thoughtfully composed. Take time with your presentation and serve with aplomb. Enjoy the praise from dinner guests and celebrate good health as you explore and cultivate your culinary creativity.

Directions: On a large serving platter or serving bowl arrange the chopped romaine. Arrange chicken, tomatoes, cucumber, feta cheese, sliced olives and red onion atop the bed of lettuce. Season the salad with salt and pepper. In a small bowl whisk together olive oil vinaigrette with the lemon juice; drizzle dressing on salad; garnish with lemon wedges.

Nutrition: Serves 4. Each serving provides 200 calories, 23 grams protein, 8 grams fat, 10 grams carbohydrate, 2 grams dietary fiber.

Try This: If you don't care for the flavor of feta cheese use crumbled goat cheese or cubed mozzarella cheese instead. ~ Look for specialty olives and pickled vegetables to add to this salad for interesting color, flavor, and texture. If pickled olives or vegetables are high in sodium place in a colander and rinse with cold running water to remove some of the salt. Drain and pat dry before adding to salad.

Chicken Salad with Tossed Romaine and Parmesan

The creamy buttermilk dressing sets this salad apart from the average making it something special and satisfying. Don't be afraid of the anchovy paste, it adds depth and flavor to a dressing that could otherwise be flat.

Ingredients for Dressing:

1/3 cup low-fat buttermilk
3 tablespoons reduced-fat mayonnaise
1 teaspoon anchovy paste
2 teaspoons Dijon-style mustard
1 tablespoon red wine vinegar
1 garlic clove, minced

Ingredients for Salad:

8 cups romaine lettuce hearts, chopped
2 cups cooked chicken, deboned, skinned, cut to 1-inch cubes
¼ cup chopped red onion
¼ cup fresh Parmesan cheese, shredded

Directions: In a small screw-top jar place the dressing ingredients. Secure top and shake well until ingredients are well mixed. Store dressing covered in the refrigerator until ready for use. Arrange chopped romaine, chicken, and chopped red onion in a large serving bowl. Just before serving toss salad with dressing coating thoroughly. Divide salad among four salad plates; season with salt and pepper; top with Parmesan cheese.

> Flavorful grainy Dijon mustard is produced on the mustard-cloaked hillsides in the Burgundy region of eastern France. Dijon mustard, named for Burgundy's capital city, is known for its clean, sharp flavor made from brown mustard seeds, white wine, unfermented grape juice and seasonings. Only mustard originating in this region may be officially labeled "Dijon". Grainy mustards similar to this regional specialty but originating elsewhere are often labeled Dijon-style.

Nutrition: Serves 4. Each serving provides 200 calories, 24 grams protein, 9 grams fat, 7 grams carbohydrate and 2 grams dietary fiber.

Try This: Consider using rotisserie chicken from your supermarket deli for any of the chicken salad recipes. Simply remove and discard the skin, take the meat off the bones and chop as directed.

Build Your Salad with These Toss-ins

☛ Indy Chef

Aiming for 21 grams of protein at lunch is a good goal and a goal we can accomplish with simple add-ins to a tossed salad. In these examples the ingredients are layered on a crisp bed of greens and the meal is ready faster than the talking box can ask, "May I take your order?" Use this as a starting point to create your personal collection of favorite 21 gram 2B/1B *Protein First* salads.

California Turkey-Avocado Toss: To your salad greens add 3 ounces diced roast turkey; 1 hard-cooked egg, diced; ¼-cup diced avocado. Dress with 1 tablespoon vinaigrette. 235 calories; 22 grams protein.

Shrimp Caesar: To salad greens add 3 ounces ready-to-eat peeled, deveined shrimp; 1 tablespoon grated Parmesan cheese; ¼-cup seasoned croutons. Dress with 1 tablespoon low-fat Caeser vinagerette. 153 calories; 21 grams protein.

I don't miss the Bun Cheeseburger Toss: To chilled salad greens add 3 ounces hot cooked crumbled ground beef, seasoned; top with 2 dill pickle chips, ¼ cup diced tomato, 1 tablespoon diced onion, and 1 ounce shredded Cheddar cheese. Dress with 1 tablespoon Thousand Island dressing. 329 calories; 24 grams protein.

Orchard Fresh Ham and Turkey Toss: Top fresh greens with 2 ounces deli-style turkey cut into cubes and 2 ounces deli-style honey-ham cut into cubes. Add ½ tart granny Smith apple, cored and diced, 1 tablespoons dried cranberries, and 1 tablespoon toasted walnuts. Dress with cider vinaigrette. 245 calories; 23 grams protein.

Lemon-Pepper Tuna Toss: Divide salad greens between two plates. Open a 4.5-ounce package Starkist® Tuna Creations Zesty Lemon Pepper and divide tuna between salads. Slice one hard-cooked egg for each salad and arrange on top of tuna. Garnish with 1 teaspoon capers, rinsed and drained. No dressing is needed. Toasted sunflower seeds are a nice addition, however. Per salad, 144 calories; 21 grams protein.

Melon, Berry and Spinach Salad with Honey Dressing

⇆ Freeway Chef, seasonal berries for sweetness, side-salad to grilled protein

This superstar summer salad is sensational included as a side dish to grilled protein. Use a variety of melon and berries taking the best your market has to offer. It is important to dress the salad with the honey and olive oil dressing: the olive oil improves the absorption of nutrients ensuring you get full health-promoting benefits from your well-chosen ingredients.

Ingredients:

8 cups spinach, washed, ready-to-eat

1 medium cantaloupe, peeled, seeded, cut into chunks

2 pints strawberries, hulled, cut in half

1 cup fresh berries, any variety

¼ cup seedless raspberry jam

¼ cup raspberry vinegar

2 tablespoons honey

2 teaspoons olive oil

¼ cup chopped macadamia nuts

Directions: In a large salad bowl gently toss the spinach, cantaloupe, strawberries, and fresh berries together. Place the jam, vinegar, honey, and oil in a jar with a tight fitting lid. Secure lid and shake vigorously for 1 minute or until emulsified. Drizzle honey dressing over spinach mixture and toss gently to coat. Top salad with macadamia nuts and serve immediately.

Calorie Burn: Shake the dressing vigorously for 1 minute to burn about the same amount of calories as you will consume from this delicious salad topper.

Food Safety: It is acceptable to refrigerate unused dressing tightly covered in mixing jar for up to 1 week. Bring to room temperature and shake well before using.

Nutrition: Serves 6: 2 cups salad per serving. Each serving provides 138 calories, 3 grams protein, 5 grams fat, 22 grams carbohydrate and 4 grams dietary fiber.

Try This: Turn this side dish into a meal by tossing diced grilled chicken breast with the melon, berries and greens. Top with freshly grated parmesan cheese. ~ For an elegant presentation cut melon using a melon baller for pretty globes of sweet summer fruit.

↪ **Freeway Chef, unexpected flavors, fancy presentation, feels like spa food**

This summertime salad showcases seasonal melons which are a good source of vitamin C, vitamin A and beta carotene. Most WLS post-ops report a good tolerance for melon and include it in their healthy weight maintenance diet.

Ingredients for Dressing:

2 tablespoons honey mustard

1 tablespoon white wine vinegar

2 teaspoons olive oil

½ teaspoon reduced-sodium soy sauce

Ingredients for Salad:

3 cups melon balls (honeydew and/or cantaloupe)

1 pound smoked turkey breast, diced

2 green onions, sliced, white parts only

2 tablespoons fresh basil leaves, torn

2 tablespoons walnuts, toasted, chopped

4 bibb lettuce leaves for garnish

Melons belong to the carotenoid family of fruits and vegetables and are rich in beta-carotene, a precursor to the fat-soluble Vitamin A. Beta-carotene is known for its antioxidant properties. It is characterized by an orange color. Carotenoid fruits include: oranges, mangoes, papayas, tomatoes, carrots, and others. Incorporate carotenoid-rich fruits and vegetables in your menu often to help promote antioxidant health.

Directions: For dressing whisk together honey mustard, white wine vinegar, olive oil and soy sauce in a small bowl. Set aside. For salad, in a large bowl toss together the melon balls, turkey, celery, green onions, basil, and walnuts. Just before serving toss salad with dressing. Serve on chilled salad plates mounding the salad in cup-shaped bibb lettuce leaves.

Nutrition: Serves 4. Each serving provides 292 calories, 33 grams protein, 13 grams fat, 12 grams carbohydrate and 1 gram dietary fiber.

Try This: When shopping for melon at your local supermarket or farmer's market select those with a smooth indentation at the stem indicating the melon was picked when it was ripe. Melon left at room temperature for a day or two becomes softer and juicier.

Melon, Tomato and Onion Salad with Goat Cheese

✿ Country Road Chef, gorgeous colors,
artful presentation, seasonal bounty

Often called a composed salad this fruit and vegetable salad is artfully arranged on the serving platter making a feast for the eyes as well as the palate. It takes time to prepare but the extra step of composing the salad goes a long way in taking your special occasion to extraordinary.

Ingredients:

1 cup sweet white onion, thinly sliced

1 cantaloupe or honeydew melon, firm but ripe

2 large tomatoes, thinly sliced

1 small cucumber, thinly sliced

½ teaspoon kosher salt

¼ teaspoon freshly ground black pepper

1 cup crumbled goat cheese

¼ cup extra-virgin olive oil

4 teaspoons balsamic vinegar

fresh basil for garnish

> "If an event is meant to matter emotionally, symbolically, or mystically, food will be close at hand to sanctify and bind it."
>
> *Diane Ackerman*

Directions: Separate onion into rings and place in a medium bowl, add cold water to cover and 1 cup of ice cubes. Set aside while preparing the other ingredients. When ready to use, drain and pat onion rings dry. Prepare melon by halving lengthwise and removing seeds and rind. Place each melon half cut-side down and slice crosswise into thin slices. Using a large round platter arrange a ring of melon slices around the edge. Top with a layer of overlapping tomato slices. Arrange a second ring of melon slices toward the center. Top with the remaining tomato slices. Tuck cucumber slices between the layers of tomato and melon. Season with kosher salt and ground black pepper: top with goat cheese and the onion rings. Drizzle with olive oil and balsamic vinegar and garnish with fresh basil leaves. Provide salad tongs for serving.

Nutrition: Serves 8. Each serving provides 165 calories, 6 grams protein, 12 grams fat, 10 grams carbohydrate, 1 gram dietary fiber.

Try This: Use this as a side dish adding more protein from another dish to meet your *Protein First* dietary needs.

Salads should contain fat, not make us fat.

I think many of us ate our way into morbid obesity by way of the salad bar. If your plate looked like mine there was an abundance of macaroni or potato salad swaddled in creamy-dreamy mayo sauce and not so much leafy greens or lean protein. And honestly, who really ever measures the dressing or better yet asks politely, "Dressing on the side, please?"

While the average salad bar continues to offer mayo sauced potatoes and pasta, these days we are likely to also see goodly offerings of lean protein, fresh organic fruits and vegetables, exotic olives, seeds, nuts, and single-serve dressing packets, made of the good fats. Studies confirm that good fats keep us feeling full longer than the no-fat or low-fat alternatives. And perhaps more importantly, good fats help our little gastric systems absorb the nutrients we eat promoting overall improved health.

Hair Health: Did you know that including healthy dietary fats in your menu leads to increased energy, soft, supple skin, and shiny, pretty hair? Aim for 20-30% of your calories to come from healthy fats. Refer to the chart on page 31.

Fish: Seafood is the best source of omega 3 fatty acids, a fat widely credited with improving cardiovascular health. Enjoy two (3-ounce) servings of cold water fish a week to lower your risk of heart attack. Include: salmon, tuna, herring, mackerel, anchovies, and sardines in your diet.

Olives and Olive Oil: The Mediterranean diet includes generous amounts of monounsaturated fats from olives and olive oil. Studies show olive oil protects the heart and appears to fight diabetes. Use dressings made of olive oil and vinegar in place of low-fat or no fat dressings; vinaigrettes are always a good choice.

Avocados: If you only look at the bottom line a serving of avocado contains as much fat as a double cheeseburger. But avocados are monounsaturated fat and including them in our diet can significantly lower unhealthy LDL cholesterol and other blood fats. Most patients of gastric surgery report a pleasing level of tolerance for avocados despite the high fat content *(many gastric patients report low tolerance for saturated fats and in some cases eating saturated fats leads to dumping syndrome.)*

Turkey Salad with Oranges and Honey-Dijon Dressing

⇆ **Freeway Chef, light and refreshing, no cooking, quick preparation**

The fresh orange sections featured in this full-meal salad brighten the turkey and enhance overall feelings of satiation. Consider this for your day-after lunch following a feasting holiday like Thanksgiving. You'll welcome the lightened change of plate.

Ingredients:

8 cups baby salad greens, ready-to-eat

12 ounces cooked turkey, chopped

1 medium sweet red pepper, cut into strips

4 oranges, peeled and sectioned

½ cup commercial honey-Dijon dressing, reduced calorie

¼ cup slivered almonds

Directions: In a large bowl toss together the salad greens, turkey, and red pepper. Divide salad mixture among four chilled salad plates. Top each salad with orange sections, 2 tablespoons of dressing and 1 tablespoon of slivered almonds.

Kaye's Choice: For ready-to-eat turkey I am partial to the Jennie-O products found in the refrigerated meat section at the market. The extra lean turkey breast comes in a variety of flavors, fully cooked, ready to cut and serve hot or cold. One (4-ounce) serving of this 98% lean protein provides 100 calories, 22 grams protein, and a trace of fat and carbohydrate. For those *"can't live without a snack"* moments enjoy a slice of turkey breast and say goodbye to hunger.

Nutrition: Serves 4. Each serving provides 281 calories, 28 grams protein, 8 grams fat, 25 grams carbohydrate and 5 grams dietary fiber.

Try This: Turkey is such a versatile protein; it lends itself to many flavors. Try including fresh berries, chopped apples or stone fruit such as peaches or nectarines in this salad. ~ For an added boost of dairy protein and calcium add one ounce of shredded or cubed cheese per serving. ~ No oranges? In a pinch 1 (11-ounce) can of mandarin oranges, drained, may be used in place of fresh oranges.

BLT Salad with Toasted Pecans

⇆ Freeway Chef, hearty and filling,
classic BLT ingredients

The bacon, lettuce and tomato sandwich – *the BLT* – is a diner classic. This salad takes the best of those flavors creating a meal that is sure to please anyone and meet our nutritional needs and weight management goals.

Ingredients:

4 slices bacon, cooked, drained, crumbled

2 teaspoons olive oil

½ cup pecans

8 cups salad greens, ready-to-eat

2 medium tomatoes, quartered

8 ounces deli-style turkey breast, sliced into strips

4 ounces Swiss cheese, ½-inch dice

½ cup Italian dressing, reduced calorie

Traditions: For centuries in Italy cooks have served the *Condijun* or *Condiglione:* a huge mixed salad and one of the few authentic main-course salads from the Italian kitchen. The salad is served in a large bowl placed in the center of the table. Diners eat directly from the bowl, creating a convivial atmosphere.

Directions: Cook bacon in a large skillet until crisp, then transfer with tongs to paper towels to drain. Pat off excess fat, crumble and set aside. Discard fat from skillet and wipe skillet clean. Heat 2 teaspoons olive oil in skillet over medium heat, add pecans and cook and stir until toasted and slightly darker in color. Transfer to paper towels to drain, season with salt and pepper and coarsely chop. In a large salad serving bowl arrange salad greens, tomatoes, turkey strips, and diced Swiss cheese. Top with crumbled bacon and toasted pecans. Serve salad with dressing on the side.

Nutrition: Serves 4. Each serving provides 353 calories, 25 grams protein, 34 grams fat, 10 grams carbohydrate and 3 grams dietary fiber.

Try This: Lighten the fat content in this salad by replacing traditional pork bacon with turkey bacon. Be sure to drain and pat dry the bacon to remove excess fat. ~ Add shredded carrots or sliced green onions to the salad greens for a change of taste and texture. ~ Bacon is a great flavor booster for salads.

Tuna and White Bean Salad

⇆ Freeway Chef, easy lunch, lasting satiation, nutritional super salad

This is a great salad on days when you need after-lunch brain power and mental stamina while curbing afternoon hunger. A Swedish study found that people who ate fish midday consumed 11% fewer calories at dinner – *that's enough to lose 8 pounds in a year* – compared with those who ate more carbs and less protein. One serving of this salad provides 33 grams protein and healthy Omega 3 fatty acids.

Ingredients for Dressing:

2 tablespoons red wine vinegar

1 tablespoon capers, rinsed and drained

1 tablespoon olive oil

½ teaspoon dried rosemary, crushed

1 small garlic clove, minced

Ingredients for Salad:

4 cups salad greens, ready-to-eat

1 (15-ounce) can great northern beans, rinsed and drained

2 (6-ounce) cans albacore tuna in water, drained, flaked with fork

2 hard-cooked eggs, coarsely chopped

¼ cup roasted red peppers, diced

> Collect a variety of flavored vinegars to enjoy in your home-crafted vinaigrettes. Look for them at gourmet food shops, farmer's markets, and at artisan and crafts fairs.

Directions: Whisk together dressing ingredients in a small bowl, set aside to allow flavors to blend. Whisk again just before dressing salad. For salad, in a large bowl toss together salad greens, beans, tuna, eggs, and red peppers. Just before serving toss with vinegar and caper dressing. Divide salad evenly among four chilled salad plates, season with salt and pepper.

Nutrition: Serves 4. Each serving provides 295 calories, 33 grams protein, 7 grams fat, 24 grams carbohydrate, 6 grams dietary fiber.

Try This: In place of canned tuna use leftover fish from the Crispy-Crusty-Crunchy Coated Protein Chapter. Cold water fish such as salmon or cod also provides healthy omega 3 fatty acids to improve brain function and promote heart health.

Black Bean and Shrimp Salsa Chunky Salad

☞ Indy Chef, light and lean,
sensational south of the border flavors

In addition to lean protein from the shrimp this salad is loaded with ridiculously healthy ingredients – and its gourmet delicious! Take advantage of ready-to-eat shrimp and prepared vegetables from the produce section to assemble this meal in short order leaving time to enjoy your meal, your companions, and your culinary brilliance.

Ingredients:

1 pound ready-to-eat medium shrimp, thawed if frozen, cut into ½-inch pieces

1 (15-ounce) can black beans, rinsed and drained

1 pint cherry tomatoes, quartered

1 large red or yellow bell pepper, chopped

1 bunch green onions, sliced, white parts only

½ cup bottled salsa

Directions: In a large mixing bowl place shrimp, black beans, cherry tomatoes, sweet bell pepper, and green onions. Add salsa and toss to coat. Allow to rest 5 to 10 minutes before serving at room temperature. Add more salsa if necessary to coat all ingredients. *Note:* since salad greens are not part of this salad the appearance should be dense, hearty and colorful; similar to a chunky chicken salad.

One 4-ounce serving of ready-to-eat shrimp has 112 calories, 24 grams protein, 1 gram fat, 0 carbohydrates. Shrimp is a low-fat protein source that provides generous amounts of B12 vitamin and niacin (B3). In addition, shrimp are rich in the iron which is a key component in enzymes and proteins, and zinc which is essential for a healthy immune system.

Nutrition: Serves 4. Each serving provides 239 calories, 31 grams protein, 2 grams fat, 22 grams carbohydrate, 8 grams dietary fiber.

Try This: Serve salad on a bed of lettuce and top with sliced avocado and a dollop of sour cream. ~ Fans of cilantro can stir-in ¼ cup chopped fresh cilantro, add a squeeze of fresh lime to enhance the flavor. ~ Consider serving this salad as a dip with toasted low-carb tortilla chips for a fun, fresh, and cleverly healthy snack alternative at your next potluck gathering.

Wilted Spinach and Tilapia Salad

⇆ Freeway Chef, simple preparation,
lean protein, vitamin rich veggies

U.S. farm-raised tilapia is a heart-healthy lean source of protein that is versatile and pairs perfectly with a variety of flavors from citrus to spice. Affordable and readily available, tilapia cooks quickly and is perfect served with fresh vegetables and salad greens.

Ingredients:

4 (4-ounce) fresh or frozen tilapia fillets

1 (6-ounce) package fresh spinach, ready-to-eat

2 tablespoons olive oil

1 (8-ounce) package fresh mushrooms, sliced

1 small yellow onion, sliced

3 cloves garlic, thinly sliced

1 large plum tomato, chopped

2 tablespoons red wine vinegar

1 teaspoon snipped fresh thyme

> "One of the very nicest things about life is the way we must regularly stop whatever it is we are doing and devote our attention to eating."
> *Luciano Pavarotti*

Directions: Thaw tilapia fillets if frozen. Preheat broiler. Season tilapia fillets with salt and pepper and arrange the fish on the unheated rack of a broiler pan sprayed with cooking spray. Broil 4-inches from the heat for 4 to 6 minutes until done. Fish will flake easily when tested with a fork: this indicates it is done. Remove fish to a plate and tent with foil to keep warm. Place spinach in a large bowl and set aside. Heat olive oil in a large skillet over medium heat: add mushrooms, onion, and garlic and cook and stir 2 to 3 minutes until tender. Stir in vinegar and cook 1 minute longer. Toss warm vegetables with spinach to slightly wilt spinach. Divide salad among four plates. Top each salad with one tilapia fillet and garnish with fresh snipped thyme. Serve immediately.

Nutrition: Serves 4. Each serving provides 213 calories, 26 grams protein, 9 grams fat, 9 grams carbohydrate, 2 grams dietary fiber.

Try This: Line the broiler catch-tray with aluminum foil before coating the rack with cooking spray: this makes clean-up a snap. ~ For wilted salad to be enjoyable the greens must be impeccably crisp and fresh before the hot protein and fat are tossed with them. Never use wilted greens to make a wilted salad.

Crab and Grapefruit Salad

⇆ Freeway Chef, no cooking required,
elegant simple supper, uncomplicated

At first glance this crab and grapefruit salad may seem extravagant but per serving it is nicely affordable, and it is quite simple to prepare. The tart-tangy grapefruit and crisp crunchy greens are a perfect foil to the sweet flavor of crabmeat.

Ingredients:

¼ cup reduced-fat mayonnaise

¼ cup peach or mango chutney

2 teaspoons Dijon-style mustard

1 (16-ounce) jar grapefruit sections, no sugar added

1 pound lump crabmeat, picked over to remove any cartilage

4 cups spring salad greens, ready-to-eat

"Food is a pleasure. It fuels us and gives us energy and the nutrients our bodies need to be replenished; rejuvenated. Take time to enjoy your food. It's one of life's greatest pleasures".
Denise Austin

Directions: Make the dressing: In a small bowl whisk together the mayonnaise, chutney, and mustard. Add 1 to 2 tablespoons of juice from the grapefruit to achieve desired consistency. Taste dressing and season with salt and pepper. Set aside. Place crabmeat in a bowl and toss with 2 tablespoons of the dressing, reserving the remaining dressing. Divide the spring salad mix among four plates. Place 5 to 6 grapefruit sections on each plate and top each salad with ¼ of the crabmeat mixture. Serve with additional dressing on the side.

Serves 4. Each serving provides 220 calories, 19 grams protein, 5 grams fat, 8 grams carbohydrate and 2 grams dietary fiber.

Try This: Look for cooked lump crabmeat in the meat section of your supermarket. This reduces the work of cooking and cleaning the crab legs and is often a better bargain. ~ Consider using imitation crabmeat in place of the lump crabmeat. ~ Fresh grapefruit may be used in place of bottled grapefruit. At the market select nice round grapefruits that feel heavy in your hand; this indicates they will be juicy. To prepare the segments carefully slice between each dividing membrane and the grapefruit pulp to release the segments. Work over a bowl to catch the juices.

Elegant Scallop and Fresh Greens Salad

Sea scallops are the larger scallops, measuring 1 to 1½-inch diameter. While they can be found fresh in the fish market they are more commonly available flash-frozen in the freezer section of your supermarket. The sweet meat is a good source of lean protein.

Ingredients:

1½ pounds sea scallops, thawed if frozen, patted dry

3 tablespoons olive oil, divided

1 tablespoons fresh chives, minced

1 tablespoon balsamic vinegar

2 garlic cloves, minced

2 teaspoons fresh tarragon, minced

2 teaspoons honey

1 teaspoon Dijon-style mustard

6 cups salad greens, ready-to-eat

1 cup shredded carrots

1 medium tomato, chopped

Benefit: The digestive system benefits from balsamic vinegar. The vinegar boosts the activity of pepsin, an enzyme that breaks down protein into smaller amino acids that can be more easily absorbed by the body, a good thing for our post-WLS nutritional needs. Pepsin helps to improve the body's metabolism as well.

Directions: Season scallops with salt and pepper on both sides. In a large skillet heat 2 tablespoons of the olive oil over medium-high heat. Add scallops and sauté until firm and opaque, turning once. Remove from skillet and keep warm. In the same skillet make dressing. Over medium heat combine remaining 1 tablespoon olive oil, chives, balsamic vinegar, garlic, tarragon, honey, and mustard. Bring to a boil and cook and stir for 30 seconds until slightly thickened. Remove from heat. Divide salad greens among four plates; top with carrots, tomato and scallops. Drizzle with dressing and serve immediately.

Nutrition: Serves 4. Each serving provides 282 calories, 30 grams protein, 12 grams fat, 14 grams carbohydrate and 2 grams dietary fiber.

Try This: For variety use large shrimp or prawns in place of the scallops.

Note:

Ingredients:

Directions:

Nutrition:

Note:

Ingredients:

Directions:

Nutrition:

feed the
carb monster soups

"Soup is easy food, easy for the eater and easy for the cook. Aside from a few basically restaurant soups, traditional and complex, a little variation in ingredients or technique will only personalize the soup rather than causing disaster."
Barbara Kafka

Feed the Carb Monster Soups

↦ **Indy Chef**   ⇄ **Freeway Chef**   ☼ **Country Road Chef**

Soups aren't *Protein First*: Should I eat them?

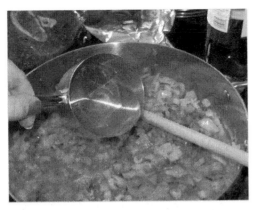

It is true, if you simply look at the nutritional line in these recipes, only half of them are *Protein First* meals. The remaining recipes contain greater amounts of carbohydrates than protein, sometimes two grams of carbohydrate to one gram of protein. Wait! Carbohydrates are those mysterious things we crave and we fear. Don't be alarmed. Before you avoid this section let's talk about why including carbohydrate soups in your post-WLS diet may be one key to avoiding weight gain down the road. Let's review the definitions:

Complex Carbohydrates: Foods that contain a lot of starch --vegetables, fruits, beans, legumes, and whole grains. They are rich in vitamins, minerals, and fiber. Foods on your plate that most closely resemble the way they come from nature, unaffected by processing, are in the complex carbohydrate group.

Simple Carbohydrates: Foods that contain a lot of sugar --*syrups, jelly, honey, soda, molasses*-- and have few, if any, vitamins and minerals and are void of fiber. Processed food including chips, crackers, cookies, cakes, pastries, and white bread are in this category.

It is popular in the health and nutrition fields to describe carbs as "good carbs" or "bad carbs". I prefer not to use those words because they assign a moral trait to food and food does not have moral traits. ***Food is food***.

Instead of good carbs and bad carbs I prefer more accurate terms:

- Fruit and Vegetable Carbs or Complex Carbs
- Grain and Starch Carbs or Complex Carbs
- Processed Manufactured Carbs or Simple Carbs

I have them arranged in nutritional importance to us after undergoing weight loss surgery. Like other nutrients carbohydrates are measured in grams. A 2008 broad-canvas study of bariatric centers revealed that few bariatric surgeons or nutritionists give a specific daily quota for carbohydrate intake. Most default to the 113 grams RDA recommended by the National Academies' Institute of Medicine for people following a 1200 calorie a day diet. It takes roughly 8 to 10 cups of fruit and vegetables to equal 113 grams complex carbohydrates and I do not know any weight loss surgery patient who can consume that much volume. Conversely, it takes less than 2 cups volume of simple carbohydrates, such as chips or cookies, to reach 113 grams of carbohydrate. When we eat simple carbohydrates we over eat. It's as well, simple, as that.

Most bariatric patients who are struggling to control their weight say they suffer from carb-cravings. We have a choice to tame those cravings: simple carbs or complex carbs, either will quiet the cravings. Simple carbs, however come without nutrients but they bring excess fat. Complex carbs are loaded with nutrients to support total wellness, plus dietary fiber we may be short of when following a high protein diet. In addition, complex carbs like to stick around and keep us full for hours. In contrast, simple carbs are a quick fix and the cravings don't stay gone for long.

We have a choice when the carb cravings hit: simple carbs or complex carbs. That is why I believe soup is a key food choice in health and weight management with weight loss surgery. Studies confirm that people who include one cup of soup in their diet each day are more likely to lose weight and sustain a healthy weight. Soup is always an intelligent choice when used as a meal or snack. I cannot think of a better way to feed the carb monster.

This chapter features the soup recipes that I include in my soup rotation. I try to always have a pot of soup in the refrigerator for snacking emergencies or a quick lunch. Soup ingredients are simple; many come from the pantry and can be kept on hand. Per serving, soup is one of the most affordable menu choices we have; many recipes call for less-expensive cuts of meat or poultry. Soups are forgiving; we can be inexact with our measurements and make substitutions more freely thus putting our signature on the recipe. If we love what we create we will look forward to eating it. These are my recipes and I hope you will use them as your platform for creativity. Here are some tips:

Measured portions: It is best to measure servings of soup to avoid over-filling the pouch and I've learned there are different ways to measure different soups. Clear soups or smooth soups without solids should be measured in 1-cup servings and eaten within about 15 minutes. Soups and stews with solids must also be measured, but differently. Use a slotted spoon to scoop solids into a 1/2-cup measuring cup. Put that in your bowl, and then add an additional 1/2-cup of the soup; both liquid and solids. This makes a good hearty 1-cup serving that should keep us full and satiated for a long time after the meal. Thick chili with beans and meat is best measured in 2/3-cup servings. It seems that these hearty dishes are much more filling and it is best to start with a smaller portion. Again, with hearty chili and stews avoid exceeding more than 1-cup volume for any meal.

Reminder: the portion size and nutritional information provided for the recipes is based on the National Academy of Sciences Recommended Daily Allowance based on a 2,000 calorie a day diet. It is expected weight loss surgery patients will eat a much smaller portion and the portion will vary by person and procedure.

Four Seasons: Often we think of soups for just fall and winter eating. I have found soups to be remarkably good year-round. The fresh produce available in spring and summer makes for terrific minestrone or garden vegetable soups. And in the summertime when I worked in an aggressively-air conditioned corporate office I found that a lunch of re-heated soup was the best antidote to the indoor chill.

The big bonus that comes from eating complex carbohydrates in soup is not calculated in weight and measure. It is the freedom from self-loathing and moral judgment that so often accompanies our food choices. In all my work with weight loss surgery patients I have never heard someone say, "I just couldn't stop eating fresh vegetables, I was out of control, I am so angry at myself for doing that." Not once. The same cannot be said for simple carbohydrate snacks that quickly become slider foods derailing our weight management.

And finally, when we eat these healthy nutrient dense soups we stay full longer and report fewer cravings for snacky-carbs. Our overall health improves, skin and hair become radiant, we maintain steady energy levels, weight management is achieved and we don't feel badly about ourselves.

Come on! Let's make soup!

Simple White Bean Soup

🏴 Indy Chef, pantry ingredients, helps
resolve Moody Pouch Syndrome (MPS)

There are days in our post WLS life when nothing sounds appealing to eat and nothing will sit well in our small stomach pouch. Keep this simple satisfying soup in mind for those days. Using convenient pantry ingredients you can prepare a soothing soup in a matter of minutes. It also travels well and reheats easily for a convenient workday lunch.

Ingredients:

1 tablespoon olive oil

½ white onion, diced

1 teaspoon Italian herb seasoning

1 (15-ounce) can great northern beans, rinsed and drained

1 (14.5-ounce) can reduced sodium chicken broth

¼ cup grated Parmesan cheese

> If you have the time use 1 cup of dried great northern beans soaked overnight in salted water. Rinse well and drain; add to soup in place of the canned beans. Simmer for 50 minutes or until beans are tender.

Directions: In a 2-quart saucepot heat olive oil over medium high heat. Add onion and cook and stir until onion is soft and translucent, about 5 minutes. Stir in Italian herb seasoning blend. Add drained great northern beans and broth. Bring to a slow simmer and continue to simmer for 5 minutes: season with salt and pepper. Ladle soup into bowls or mugs and top each serving with 1 tablespoon Parmesan cheese.

If a soup puree is desired, after soup has simmered 5 minutes use an immersion blender to puree soup or blend soup in batches in blender, returning to pot to keep warm.

Nutrition: Serves 3. Each 1-cup serving provides 253 calories, 19 grams protein, 8 grams fat, 32 grams carbohydrate, 7 grams dietary fiber.

Try This: To include more vegetables sauté a diced carrot and one stalk of sliced celery with the onion. ~ In place of the Italian herb seasoning use 1 or 2 tablespoons of fresh pesto to flavor your soup. ~ Make a double batch for a family meal; serve with crusty bread.

☼ **Country Road Chef, guilt-free comfort food, crowd friendly**

This famous soup, which is served daily by decree of law in the United States Senate lunchroom, is hearty and comforting. It fits our ☼ Country Road Chef criteria because preparing the beans by soaking is an overnight process. The actual cooking method is uncomplicated as is the soup.

Ingredients:

1 pound dried navy beans

3 quarts cold water

1 tablespoon canola oil

1 tablespoon butter

3 medium onions, diced

4 stalks celery, finely chopped

3 cloves garlic, minced

1 (1-2 pound) ham bone with meat

2 (48-ounce) cans chicken broth, reduced-sodium

¼ cup fresh parsley, finely chopped

Navy beans are small white legumes, also called Yankee beans. Because of their nutritional value and long storage life, the United States Navy has served these healthy beans regularly since the mid-1800's, and from there comes the name. Affordable dried navy beans are delicious in soups, salads, and baked bean dishes.

Directions: Place beans in a large Dutch oven and cover with the 3 quarts cold water: let sit overnight. Drain and rinse beans. Set aside. In the same Dutch oven heat the canola oil and butter over medium high heat. Add the onion and celery and cook until soft and translucent, about 10 minutes. Add the garlic and cook 3 minutes. Place the ham bone in the pot. Return the soaked beans to the pot and add the chicken broth. Bring soup to a low boil, reduce heat to a low simmer; cover and cook 90 minutes, stirring occasionally. Test beans for doneness: they should be tender to bite but still hold their shape. Remove ham bone and allow to cool: pull meat from ham bone and return meat to pot. Discard bone. Season the soup with salt and pepper. Stir in chopped parsley just before serving.

Nutrition: Serves 10. Each 1-cup serving provides 283 calories, 27 grams protein, 11 grams fat, 19 grams carbohydrate, 4 grams dietary fiber.

Split Pea Soup

Split peas are an abundant source of fiber and protein, and they also supply good amounts of potassium and the B vitamin, folate. Split peas are available in green or yellow and they are affordable.

Ingredients:

2 tablespoons canola oil

2 large carrots, thinly sliced

2 large celery stalks, thinly sliced

1 bay leaf

1 tablespoon Old Bay® Seafood Seasoning

1 (16-ounce) package dry split peas, green or yellow, rinsed and picked over

1 (1-2 pound) ham bone or 3-4 smoked ham hocks

2 (14.5-ounce) cans reduced sodium vegetable broth

2 cups water

Directions: In a large Dutch oven or stockpot heat the canola oil over medium high heat. Add the carrots and celery and cook and stir 5 minutes. Add the bay leaf and Old Bay® Seafood Seasoning and stir to combine. Add the split peas, ham bone, vegetable broth, and water. Bring to a gentle boil. Reduce heat to low; cover; simmer 1 hour. Remove ham bone to cutting board; cut off meat and discard bone. Cut meat into bite-sized chunks and return to soup. Remove and discard bay leaf. Season the soup with salt and pepper. Serve warm.

Alternative slow cooker method: Omit canola oil and the step of sautéing the carrots and celery. Place all ingredients in slow cooker: cover; set to low and cook for 8-10 hours or high and cook for 4 to 6 hours. Follow steps described above beginning with removing the ham bone.

Nutrition: Serves 6. Each 1½-cup serving provides 368 calories, 29 grams protein, 11 grams fat, 20 grams carbohydrate, 7 grams dietary fiber.

Try This: For a creamy split pea soup stir-in 1 (12-ounce) can evaporated milk in the last 15 minutes of cooking.

Sun-Dried Tomato Soup

Sun-dried tomatoes have been placed in the sun to remove most of the water content from them. In the process they keep their nutritional value and are high in lycopene, and vitamin C. For this recipe use sun dried tomatoes that are packaged dry, not in olive oil.

Ingredients:

2 teaspoons olive oil

½ cup red onion, finely chopped

1 stalk celery, finely chopped

1 medium carrot, peeled, finely chopped

1 teaspoon dried basil

1 teaspoon dried thyme

1 bay leaf

1 (6-ounce) can tomato paste

1 (48-ounce) can reduced sodium chicken broth

3 ounces sun-dried tomatoes, chopped

1 clove garlic, minced

1 tablespoon honey

Tomato paste, available in cans and tubes, consists of slow cooked tomatoes that are reduced to a deep red, concentrate. Tomato paste contains the antioxidant lycopene which may reduce the risk of some cancers. Studies suggest tomato consumption may be beneficial in reducing the risk of cardiovascular illness associated with type 2 diabetes.

Directions: In a large Dutch oven or stockpot heat olive oil. Add onion, celery, and carrot and sauté for 2-3 minutes. Stir in the basil, thyme, bay leaf, tomato paste and 1 cup of the broth. Stir and cook until well mixed. Add the remaining broth, the chopped sun-dried tomatoes, minced garlic, and honey. Bring soup to a boil then lower heat to a simmer. Cover and cook at a simmer for 1 hour. Remove and discard bay leaf, season soup with salt and pepper. Serve warm.

Nutrition: Serves 6. Each 1½-cup serving provides 60 calories, 2 grams protein, 2 grams fat, 10 grams carbohydrate, 3 grams dietary fiber.

Try This: Top with freshly grated Cheddar or Parmesan cheese. ~ Try using fresh herbs in place of the dried herbs for summer-like flavor.

Tomato and Cheese Tortellini Soup

⚑ Indy Chef, fast and easy, multiple
flavor enhancing options

This simple soup made from pantry ingredients is a good answer to those pasta cravings we invariably get after weight loss surgery. The tortellini is served in controlled portions as part of the soup which helps prevent over-consumption of the soft simple carbohydrate. While this recipe falls short in protein it does serve the purpose of taming carb and pasta cravings in a well-reasoned manner, as well as delivering nutrients including vitamins and minerals.

Ingredients:

1 (14.5-ounce) can diced tomatoes with roasted garlic and onion

1 (14.5-ounce) can reduced sodium chicken broth

1 (12-ounce) package fresh cheese tortellini

1 small zucchini, sliced

¼ cup Parmesan cheese, grated

> "One way to motivate yourself is to recognize how gratifying it is to make a goal, identify the specific steps to get there, follow your plan, and reap the rewards."
> Judith J. Wurtman

Directions: In a large 3-quart saucepot combine diced tomatoes and chicken broth; bring to a boil. Cover, reduce heat and simmer 5 minutes. Add ravioli and zucchini; bring to a boil. Cover, reduce heat, and simmer 8-10 minutes or until ravioli and zucchini are tender. Season the soup with salt and pepper. Serve warm topped with grated Parmesan cheese.

Nutrition: Serves 4. Each 1¼-cup serving provides 317 calories, 14 grams protein, 6 grams fat, 38 grams carbohydrate, 1 gram dietary fiber.

Try This: Look for different varieties of canned tomatoes to change the flavor of your soups. Try diced with roasted garlic and onion; petite diced with chipotle chiles; or diced with basil, garlic and oregano. ~ A cup of soup is always a smart choice for a snack because it satiates our craving for carbohydrate and delivers readily absorbed nutrients.

Autumn Vegetable Minestrone

✿ Country Road Chef, nutritious
homemade comfort food

Preparing the vegetables for this soup takes time and should be enjoyed as part of the act of creating a nutritious and delicious meal for those lucky enough to join you at your table. Enjoy the journey to the destination.

Ingredients:

¼ cup olive oil

2 cloves garlic, minced

1 medium white onion, cut into ½-inch dice

1 medium carrot, peeled, thinly sliced

1 stalk celery with leaves, thinly sliced

1 (8-ounce) package button mushrooms, sliced

8 plum (roma) tomatoes, peeled, seeded, chopped

6 ounces fresh green beans cut to 1-inch lengths

2 cups pumpkin or butternut squash, peeled and cut into ½-inch cubes

½ green cabbage, thinly sliced

1 (15-ounce) can kidney beans, rinsed and drained

2 (14.5-ounce) cans reduced sodium vegetable broth

4 cups water

1½ cups uncooked medium seashell pasta

¼ cup fresh basil, chopped

Directions: In a large stockpot heat the olive oil over medium high heat. Add the garlic, onion, carrot, celery, and mushrooms and cook and stir until the vegetables sweat and start to soften, about 5 minutes. Add the tomatoes, green beans, pumpkin or butternut squash, cabbage, kidney beans, vegetable broth, and water. Bring to a boil and then lower heat to maintain a slow simmer. Cover and cook soup 2 hours, stirring occasionally. Return soup to a gentle boil and stir-in seashell pasta: cook for 12 minutes or until pasta is done. Stir in fresh basil and serve warm.

Nutrition: Serves 8. Each 1½-cup serving provides 252 calories, 12 grams protein, 8 grams fat, 37 grams carbohydrate, 7 grams dietary fiber.

Grandma's Mushroom Barley Soup

⇆ Freeway Chef, one pot meal,
nutritional superstar soup

This soup featuring fresh mushrooms and pearl barley will not only tame the hungriest carb monster, it provides nutrients that promote good health. Mushrooms contain compounds which inhibit the formation of cancerous tumors, and pearl barley is a cholesterol-lowering soluble fiber.

Ingredients:

2 teaspoons canola oil

1 tablespoon butter, unsalted

1 onion, finely chopped

2 cloves garlic, minced

2 carrots, peeled, finely chopped

2 stalks celery, with leafy tops, finely chopped

½ pound white button mushrooms, trimmed and thinly sliced

½ pound fresh shiitake mushrooms, trimmed, thinly sliced

¼ teaspoon nutmeg, freshly grated

1 (14.5-ounce) can vegetable broth, reduced sodium

1 (14.5-ounce) can stewed tomatoes

1 cup water

½ cup pearled barley

The high fiber content in this soup makes it a smart dish to include in a *Protein First* diet. Barley contains soluble fiber similar to oatmeal, and is believed to contribute to lowered cholesterol levels thus promoting heart health.

Directions: In a large 4-quart Dutch oven heat canola oil and butter over medium high heat. Add onion and garlic and cook 2 to 3 minutes until vegetables start to sweat. Add carrots, celery, and mushrooms to pot; cook and stir 8 to 10 minutes allowing vegetables to cook and release juices. Grate fresh nutmeg over vegetables and season with salt and pepper. Add vegetable broth, stewed tomatoes, and water. Bring to a boil. Reduce heat to simmer, cover, and cook 30 minutes. Stir in pearl barley and simmer uncovered 30 minutes or until the barley is tender. If soup becomes too thick add additional broth or water, ½ cup at a time until desired thickness is achieved. Serve warm.

Nutrition: Serves 6. Each 1½-cup serving provides 268 calories, 10 grams protein, 4 grams fat, 54 grams carbohydrate, 10 grams dietary fiber.

Beef Vegetable Soup with Barley

⇆ Freeway Chef, low-maintenance preparation, excellent for leftovers

This hearty soup provides a sensible balance of succulent beef protein with tender vegetables. For WLS patients that have trouble tolerating beef this is a good recipe to try because the moist simmering renders the meat tender and succulent.

Ingredients:

3 tablespoons canola oil

1½ pounds beef stew meat, cubed

5 large carrots, peeled, sliced

5 medium celery stalks, sliced

2 large mild onions, diced

8 ounces button mushrooms, sliced

10 cups water

1 cup pearled barley

1 teaspoon dried oregano

2 tablespoons beef bouillon granules

The popularity of canola oil is growing in the United States, in light of news about its health benefits. Canola oil, expressed from rape seeds, contains cholesterol-balancing monounsaturated fat, similar to olive oil. In addition, it contains omega 3 fatty acids which lower cholesterol and triglycerides while supporting brain function. The bland taste makes it more suitable than olive oil in many dishes where the flavor of the oil should go undetected.

Directions: In a large 4-quart Dutch oven or stockpot heat the canola oil over medium high heat. Season the beef stew meat with salt and pepper and add to hot oil, cooking and stirring until browned. Remove beef to plate, set aside. To the hot drippings add carrots, celery, onions, and mushrooms. Cook and stir the vegetables until they soften and start to brown. Return beef to pot. Add water, barley, oregano and bouillon granules. Bring to a boil. Reduce heat to simmer, cover, and cook stirring occasionally for 90 minutes. Serve warm

Nutrition: Serves 8. Each 1½-cup serving provides 322 calories, 22 grams protein, 13 grams fat, 29 grams carbohydrate, 7 grams dietary fiber.

Try This: Add a variety of vegetables to this soup making the most of fresh ingredients and seasonal favorites. ~ Top each serving with shredded Cheddar cheese for added flavor and dairy nutrients.

Chicken and Barley Soup

⇆ **Freeway Chef, a better chicken soup, ideal for cold and flu season**

Keep this soup in mind when cold and flu season is at hand. The healing nutrients and emotional comfort in a carefully crafted cup of chicken soup can never be underestimated. Serve yourself or a loved one a warm cup at the first sign of sniffles and let the cozy old-fashioned healing begin.

Ingredients:

1 pound boneless skinless chicken breasts cut into 1-inch cubes

2 tablespoons canola oil

2 medium shallots, diced

2 stalks celery, with leafy tops, thinly sliced

2 carrots, peeled, thinly sliced

1 (8-ounce) package button mushrooms, sliced

1 clove garlic, minced

2 (14.5-ounce) cans chicken broth, reduced sodium

2 cups water

1 bay leaf

½ teaspoon dried thyme

½ cup pearled barley

> "It's difficult to think anything but pleasant thoughts while eating a comforting bowl of warm homemade chicken soup."
> *Lewis Goddard*

Directions: In a large 4-quart Dutch oven heat the canola oil over medium high heat. Brown the chicken pieces turning to cook on all sides. Remove to plate and set aside. Keeping the Dutch oven over medium high heat add the diced shallot, celery, carrots, mushrooms and garlic. Cook for 6 to 8 minutes until vegetables brown and start to become tender. Return chicken to pot with juices. Add broth, water, bay leaf, and thyme. Bring to a boil. Reduce heat; cover and simmer for 15 minutes. Return soup to a boil and stir in barley. Again, reduce heat to simmer and cook 15 minutes until barley is tender. Discard bay leaf and serve immediately.

Nutrition: Serves 6. Each 1½-cup serving provides 218 calories, 21 grams protein, 7 grams fat, 19 grams carbohydrate, 4 grams dietary fiber.

Try This: If you prefer dark meat chicken use boneless skinless chicken thighs in place of the breast meat.

⇆ Freeway Chef, big spicy flavor,
convenient ingredients

This colorful and flavorful soup comes together quicker than you can say taco take-out. The traditional flavors of Mexican food are showcased in this nutrition-packed soup. This is a fine use for leftover chicken or turkey.

Ingredients:

1 tablespoon canola oil

1 large onion, chopped

1 large red sweet pepper, seeded, chopped

1½ teaspoons chili powder

1 teaspoon ground cumin

2 (14.5-ounce) cans reduced sodium chicken broth

2 cups water

1 (14.5-ounce) can Mexican-style stewed tomatoes

1 (15-ounce) can black beans, rinsed and drained

1 (8-ounce) package butternut squash, cut to ½-inch dice

2 cups cooked chopped chicken meat, boneless, skinless

1 cup frozen whole kernel corn

¼ cup fresh cilantro, chopped or ¼ cup fresh parsley, chopped

Directions: In a large 4-quart Dutch oven heat canola oil over medium high heat. Add onion, red pepper, chili powder, and ground cumin and cook about 5 minutes until tender. Add chicken broth, water, and tomatoes. Bring to a boil. Add black beans, squash, chicken, and corn and return to boil. Lower heat to a simmer, cover, and cook 20 minutes. Stir in cilantro or parsley and serve immediately.

Nutrition: Serves 6. Each 1½-cup serving provides 267 calories, 27 grams protein, 6 grams fat, 29 grams carbohydrate, 7 grams dietary fiber.

Try This: In place of the stewed tomatoes use a 16-ounce jar of your favorite salsa. ~ Garnish soup with a dollop of sour cream, chopped fresh avocado, shredded cheese, or sliced fresh green onions.

Chicken and Soba Noodle Soup

⇆ Freeway Chef, international flavor, simple preparation, nutrient dense

While the ingredient list seems long, this Indonesian inspired soup comes together quickly. Prepare all ingredients before beginning the cooking process and enjoy this fresh soup with healthy whole grain soba noodles.

Ingredients:

1 tablespoon canola oil

1 medium yellow onion, sliced

2 tablespoons fresh ginger, grated

2 cups napa cabbage, shredded

2 stalks celery, thinly sliced

4 cups water

2 tablespoons chicken bouillon granules

1 tablespoon reduced sodium soy sauce

½ teaspoon crushed red pepper flakes

1 pound cooked chicken, light and dark meat, chopped

1 (8-ounce) package whole grain soba noodles

4 green onions, chopped, white parts only

juice of 1 lime

¼ cup unsalted dry-roasted peanuts, chopped

Cooking the soba noodles separately from the soup allows us to control portion size. In addition, the noodles stay tender, retaining their hearty buckwheat flavor. Soba noodles have a long shelf life; include them in your standard pantry inventory.

Directions: Heat canola oil in a large stockpot over high heat. Add onion and ginger and cook, stirring constantly until onion begins to brown and becomes aromatic. Add cabbage and celery and continue stir-fry cooking for 4 minutes. Add water, bouillon granules, soy sauce, and red pepper flakes. Bring to a boil; reduce heat to simmer. Add chicken, cover and simmer 15 minutes. Meanwhile, cook soba noodles following package directions, set aside and keep warm. Remove soup from heat, stir in green onions and lime juice. Serve 1 cup of soup over 1/3 cup cooked soba noodles. Garnish with chopped peanuts.

Nutrition: Serves 6. Each serving provides 305 calories, 30 grams protein, 6 grams fat, 33 grams carbohydrate, 2 grams dietary fiber.

⇆ Freeway Chef, bright lemon flavor,
quality protein, nutritious veggies

This is a fresh take on chicken soup with the added nutritional benefit of eggs and the fresh flavor of lemon. Good any time of the year.

Ingredients:

1 teaspoon olive oil

1 small clove garlic, minced

6 cups chicken broth, reduced sodium

1 rib celery, chopped

1 cup shredded carrots

½ teaspoon ground black pepper

¼ teaspoon salt

½ cup orzo (small-grain pasta)

2½ cups frozen green peas or green beans

3 cups chopped cooked chicken

2 large eggs

3-4 tablespoons freshly squeezed lemon juice (about 1 large lemon)

SNAP!

*Pictured on
Front Cover*

Directions: Heat olive oil in a Dutch oven over medium heat. Add garlic and cook until light brown, about 1 minute. Add broth, celery, carrots, pepper, and salt and bring to a boil over high heat. Add orzo and reduce heat to a simmer. Cook until orzo is tender, about 8 minutes. Add peas and chicken and simmer 2 minutes. (Note: If freezing portions of this soup do so at this step, before adding eggs. Add eggs to thawed soup in final stage of reheating.) Meanwhile whisk eggs and 3 tablespoons of the lemon juice in medium bowl. Temper egg mixture by slowly whisking in about 1 cup hot broth in a thin stream. Whisk egg mixture into soup and warm briefly over low heat, 2 minutes. Do not boil or eggs will curdle. Adjust seasoning to taste with lemon juice, salt, and pepper and serve.

Nutrition: Per 1 cup serving: 212 calories, 25 grams protein, 5 grams fat, 16 grams carbohydrate (2 grams dietary fiber).

Try This: Add 1 tablespoon grated fresh ginger to soup with the garlic. Garlic and ginger are immunity boosters and will help the body fight colds and infection.

Italian Sausage Soup

Enjoy the fresh spicy flavors of pizza in an easy to prepare soup. This soup reheats well for a filling mid-day meal.

Ingredients:

2 teaspoons canola oil

1 clove garlic, minced

1 medium onion, diced

1 teaspoon Italian seasoning

1 pound lean ground turkey

8 ounces premium pork Italian sausage*

2 (14.5-ounce) cans reduced sodium beef broth

2 (14.5-ounce) can Italian-style stewed tomatoes, undrained

2 large carrots, sliced ¼-inch thick

1 (15-ounce) can great northern beans, rinsed and drained

2 small zucchini, halved lengthwise, sliced

2 cups baby spinach, washed, ready-to-eat

Enjoy leftover Italian Sausage Soup by reheating in the microwave following food safety guidelines. Because microwaves heat unevenly the soup must be stirred mid-way through heating. It is important that soup temperature is 165°F before eating to destroy any food borne illness. After reaching correct temperature allow the soup to rest and cool slightly before eating. See the Safe Minimum Cooking Temperatures chart on page 181.

Directions: In a large 4-quart stockpot heat canola oil over medium high heat. Add garlic, onion and Italian seasoning; sauté until onion begins to soften and turn golden brown. Add the ground turkey and Italian sausage and break up with wooden spoon as it browns. Cook until well browned; add beef broth and stewed tomatoes. Bring to boil, reduce heat to simmer. Add carrots, great northern beans, and zucchini. Cover and simmer 15 minutes or until zucchini is tender. Remove from heat, add the spinach and stir. Replace lid and keep covered for 5 minutes while spinach cooks. Serve warm. *I prefer Jimmy Dean® Premium Pork Italian Sausage.

Nutrition: Serves 8. Each 1½-cup serving provides 460 calories, 31 grams protein, 18 grams fat, 45 grams carbohydrate, 13 grams dietary fiber.

Try This: Top soup with a generous serving of grated mozzarella cheese for a meal celebrating the fresh taste of Italy. ~ Mix together ground turkey and sausage, shape into small meatballs, broil in oven, and add to soup.

Zesty Hamburger Soup

Spicy V8® juice takes this ordinary hamburger soup to spicy goodness that is a crowd pleaser and WLS friendly. Serve this at your next tailgate party.

Ingredients:

1 tablespoon canola oil

2 stalks celery, sliced ½-inch thick

1 medium onion, diced

1 clove garlic, minced

2 pounds extra lean ground beef

2 cups frozen whole kernel corn

1 (4-ounce) can diced green chiles

4 cups V8® Spicy Hot vegetable juice

4 cups water

2 (14.5-ounce) cans diced tomatoes

1 (15-ounce) can black beans, rinsed and drained

2 cups small shell pasta, uncooked

8 ounces Cheddar cheese, shredded

Soup has been a part of the American diet since colonial times. In that era soup was valued as an energy restorative and the first colonial cookbook published in 1742 included several soup recipes. It wasn't until 140 years later that the first pamphlet dedicated to soup recipes was published in 1882: Soups and Soup Making by Emma Ewing. Today there are more than 1,100 cookbooks dedicated to soup in print. A recent study showed, however, that 68 percent of home cooks do not follow a recipe when making soup.

Directions: In a large Dutch oven heat canola oil over medium high heat. Add celery, onion, and garlic; cook 5 minutes. Add ground beef and cook, breaking apart meat as it cooks; season with salt and pepper. Add whole kernel corn, diced green chiles, V8® juice, water, tomatoes, and beans. Bring to a boil. Reduce heat to simmer, cover and cook 20 minutes. Increase heat and bring soup to boil; add uncooked shell pasta. Stir and cook 12 minutes or until pasta is done. Serve warm topped with Cheddar.

Nutrition: Serves 8. Each 2-cup serving provides 473 calories, 28 grams protein, 22 grams fat, 41 grams carbohydrate, 5 grams dietary fiber.

Try This: Prepare this meal in your slow cooker. Simply brown the ground beef in a skillet, place browned meat in slow cooker with all ingredients except pasta, cover; cook on low 6 to 8 hours or high 2 to 4 hours. Add pasta in final hour of cooking.

Chipotle Meatballs and Veggie Soup

⇆ Freeway Chef, exciting vibrant
contrasting flavors, company friendly

This simple meatball soup surprises with the unexpected smoky flavor of chipotle. Adjust the heat by changing the amount of chipotle in adobo sauce that you incorporate into the meatballs.

Ingredients:

2 tablespoons canola oil

1 small onion, diced

4 carrots, sliced ½-inch thick

2 stalks celery, sliced ½-inch thick

2 (14.5-ounce) cans reduced sodium chicken broth

1 (15-ounce) can hominy, rinsed and drained

2 cups water

1 pound lean ground pork

1 large egg

¼ cup plain bread crumbs

½ to 1-tablespoon chipotles in adobo sauce, chopped

juice of 1 lime, plus lime wedges for garnish

> The contrast of smoky chipotle with fresh lime juice awakens the taste buds. Eating and enjoying a variety of interesting flavors is essential to preventing post-meal cravings, and ultimately a contributing factor to our weight maintenance success.

Directions: In a large stockpot heat the olive oil over medium heat. Add the onion, carrots, and celery: season vegetables with a pinch of salt and pinch of white sugar; cook, stirring occasionally until vegetables are tender. Add broth, hominy, and water. Bring to a simmer. Meanwhile, heat oven to 425°F and line a rimmed baking sheet with foil, coat with cooking spray. In a medium bowl combine the pork, egg, bread crumbs, chipotles, and a pinch of salt. Form the pork mixture into 20 meatballs, 1 tablespoon each. Place on prepared baking sheet and bake in preheated oven 14 to 16 minutes, until done. Keep soup at a low simmer while meatballs bake. Add the cooked meatballs to soup and stir-in lime juice. Remove from heat; serve soup garnished with lime wedges.

Nutrition: Serves 5. Each 1½-cup serving provides 328 calories, 28 grams protein, 15 grams fat, 28 grams carbohydrate, 4 grams dietary fiber.

Hot and Sour Pork Soup

This is classic hot and sour soup, a Chinese take-out favorite. The fresh ginger adds its distinct sweet peppery flavor and pairs with the rice vinegar to aid digestion.

Ingredients:

¼ cup dried porcini or other dried mushrooms

1 cup boiling water

2 tablespoons soy sauce, reduced sodium

1 tablespoon cornstarch

1 teaspoon dark brown sugar

1 (1-pound) pork tenderloin, thinly sliced, cut into thin strips

2 teaspoons canola oil

¼ teaspoon red pepper flakes

1 (8-ounce) package button mushrooms, sliced

4 green onions, thinly sliced, whites and greens

1 (14.5-ounce) can reduced sodium chicken broth

¼ cup rice vinegar or cider vinegar

2 tablespoons tomato paste

1 (1-inch) piece fresh ginger, grated, juices reserved

¼ teaspoon cayenne pepper

Directions: Place dried porcini mushrooms in a small bowl, cover with boiling water, set aside. In a medium non-reactive bowl whisk together soy sauce, cornstarch, and brown sugar; add sliced pork and toss to coat, set aside to marinate. Once porcini mushrooms have hydrated, about 20 minutes, scoop from the water, rinse, and thinly slice. Strain the soaking water through a fine-mesh sieve or colander lined with a paper coffee filter: reserve liquid, discard solids. In a large 3-quart saucepan heat the canola oil over medium heat. Add the red pepper flakes, button mushrooms, and green onions. Cook, stirring, until mushrooms are soft; add chicken broth, porcini mushrooms, vinegar, tomato paste, ginger with reserved juice, cayenne, and reserved mushroom soaking liquid. Bring to a boil; reduce heat to a simmer; cover and simmer 10 minutes. Increase heat and bring to a boil, add the marinated pork and cook at low boil uncovered 4 to 6 minutes, until pork is done and soup is slightly thickened. Serve warm.

Nutrition: Serves 4. Each serving provides 231 calories, 31 grams protein, 6 grams fat, 14 grams carbohydrate, 2 grams dietary fiber.

Green Chili with Spicy Pork Tenderloin

✿ Country Road Chef, traditional green chili, savory slow-cooked flavor

This traditional green chili with pork is perfect for taking the chill off a cool autumn afternoon. Look for a variety of fresh chile peppers available seasonally at the Farmer's Market and roadside vegetable stands. You may be able to find chiles that have been smoked, saving you this step.

Ingredients:

3 fresh Anaheim chile peppers

2 tablespoons canola oil

1½ pounds lean pork tenderloin, cut to 1-inch cubes

2 large onions, chopped

3 cloves garlic, minced

1 (28-ounce) can tomatillos, chopped

1 (15-ounce) can navy beans, rinsed and drained

1 tablespoon ground cumin

2 teaspoons dried oregano, crushed

4 cups water

2 tablespoons vegetable bouillon granules

juice of 1 lime

¼ cup fresh cilantro, chopped

"Cooking is part work, part play. It is also common sense, and can be a form of self-expression. Recipes bear the mark of the person making them, not just the person writing them. I hope that you will feel the freedom to experiment a little or even a lot with them."

Jenna Holst - Stews

Directions: Preheat oven to 400°F. Arrange chile peppers on a foil-lined baking sheet coated with cooking spray. Roast 25 to 30 minutes or until skins are dark, turning once halfway through roasting. Place chile peppers in a bowl; cover with plastic wrap and let stand 10 minutes. Carefully remove skins, stems, and seeds; chop chile peppers; set aside. In a large stockpot heat canola oil over medium high heat; add pork, cook until browned. Add onions and garlic; continue cooking until onions are tender, stirring occasionally. Stir in chopped roasted chile peppers, tomatillos, navy beans, ground cumin, oregano, water, and bouillon granules. Bring to a boil, reduce heat, simmer covered for 40 minutes. Remove from heat, stir in lime juice and chopped cilantro. Serve warm.

Nutrition: Serves 6. Each 1½-cup serving provides 304 calories, 32 grams protein, 8 grams fat, 26 grams carbohydrate, 10 grams dietary fiber.

Turkey Chili

Fresh ground turkey is increasingly available at major supermarkets. For the leanest preparation select all white meat ground turkey.

Ingredients:

1 tablespoon canola oil

1 medium onion, diced

2 cloves garlic, minced

1 each yellow and red bell pepper, diced

2 teaspoons chili powder

1 teaspoon salt-free Mexican seasoning blend

1 pound lean ground turkey

1 (15-ounce) can red kidney beans, rinsed and drained

1 (14.5-ounce) can stewed tomatoes

1 (8-ounce) can tomato sauce

2 tablespoons tomato paste

2 tablespoons jalapeño jelly or 2 tablespoons brown sugar

Poultry should be fully cooked to destroy the bacteria that could cause food borne illness. The correct safe cooking temperature will be stated on the package; measure with a meat thermometer. Never eat under-cooked poultry.

Ground turkey must be cooked to well-done: 165°F. See Safe Minimum Cooking Temperatures chart on page 181.

Directions: Heat canola oil in a large stockpot over medium high heat. Add onion, garlic, and bell peppers. Cook and stir until vegetables start to sweat and become tender. Add chili powder and seasoning blend. Add ground turkey, cook and stir, breaking apart as it cooks. When turkey is completely browned add kidney beans, stewed tomatoes, tomato sauce, tomato paste, and jalapeño jelly or brown sugar. Reduce heat and simmer for 20 minutes. Note: if chili is too thick add water or chicken broth to achieve desired consistency. Serve warm.

Nutrition: Serves 4. Each 2-cup serving provides 321 calories, 37 grams protein, 6 grams fat, 44 grams carbohydrate, 10 grams dietary fiber.

Try This: Prepare a variety of condiments to top chili including sour cream, shredded cheese, chopped onion, diced avocado. ~ For a taco salad serve chili atop shredded lettuce and garnished with broken tortilla chips.

My Favorite Feed the Carb Monster Soup:

Note:

Ingredients:

Directions:

Nutrition:

crispy crusty CRUNCHY COATED Protein

"I'm happiest when sitting down to a good meal with people I know well, the food is not being worshiped or fawned over, but rather has just simply taken its natural place in the moment. The message that comes across to the friends gathered at the table is that, yes, delicious food is important, but just as important are good times involved with the sharing of that food."
Gordon Hamersley

Crispy Crusty Crunchy Coated Protein

↜ **Indy Chef**   ⇆ **Freeway Chef**   ✿ **Country Road Chef**

Something Crunchy From My Oven Comes

Have you found yourself craving something crisp and crunchy when following the WLS high protein diet? It is common when a diet is void of satisfying crunchy foods to crave crispy textures and the savory salty flavors associated with crunchy food. When we fight these cravings it is only so long before we surrender --*I can't take it anymore*-- and dip into the chip bag or cracker barrel for temptingly available effortless crunch. But we know this is detrimental to our WLS diet because the empty carbs are easily converted to body fat. In addition we tend to eat snacking carbs with liquids thus turning them into slider foods which fail to fill the stomach pouch and produce feelings of satiation.

Quite by chance I discovered that crisp coated protein baked in the oven is a remarkably satisfying means to solving the crunch craving crisis. In addition, a meal centered on a crispy oven-fried protein is family friendly and wildly popular without ever tasting like diet food. And there is no better canvas for flavor enhancement and experimentation than the basic crumb coating. Creative flavors add variety and personalization to an otherwise ordinary dish. Most importantly, crispy coated protein is a terrific way to stay on course with our health and dietary goals.

This chapter teaches how to prepare our ordinary protein wrapped in a crispy crunchy crust. I've been experimenting with crispy-cooking for many years and this is the best of what I have learned. I hope you will find room on your plate for something crunchy!

Crispy Crunchy Oven-Fried Protein: The Method

Rack Roasting: The first challenge for us is to create a crisp coating without deep frying in oil. Eating deep fried food may cause dumping syndrome and the extra calories added during cooking may ultimately lead to weight gain. A better cooking method for us is rack roasting in the oven. This method is employed in several of the recipes in this section and it is easy to accomplish. First, cover a rimmed baking sheet (a cookie sheet) with foil, shiny side up. Next place a wire cooling rack (the kind used for cooling cakes and cookies) on the baking sheet atop the foil. Spray the rack with cooking spray and place coated protein on the rack to bake according to recipe directions. This method prevents the bottom of the protein from over-crusting or caramelizing which happens if it is placed directly on the baking sheet.

Position crumb coated protein evenly spaced and not touching. Clean-up is a snap: after cooling discard the aluminum foil and scrub the rack with sudsy warm water. The health benefits of this method are stellar! When compared to deep-fried chicken, rack-roasted chicken contains about 40-percent less fat. There's a crunch we can enjoy.

Crust Coating: Next, in order to achieve a perfect crunch with rack roasting, we need to proceed with a different breading method than we would with deep frying. The traditional breading method practiced by our mothers and grandmothers and by most home cooks today is to dust the protein in flour, dip in a liquid solution of whisked eggs and milk, and coat in a seasoned crumb mixture of flour, bread crumbs, ground crackers, cornmeal or the like. Some very good fried chicken and crusty fish has come of this method. But the results can be unpredictable: the protein from the flour, eggs, and milk can toughen the crust and absorb too much of the cooking fat. The crust can become soggy and fall flat if not well-seasoned. I know this from experience - *some very disappointing experience*. In my quest for the perfect crave-curbing crunch I studied many cookbooks, culinary textbooks, and spoke with professional chefs. With a few changes to the traditional process and predictable ingredients I am happy to report my crust has crunch – and yours will too.

Step 1: Dusting
Cornstarch: Replace the dusting flour with cornstarch. Traditionally, the first step in crusting is to dredge the protein in flour. But flour contains proteins (gluten) which mix with moisture from the meat and the dipping solution creating a heavy, sometimes gummy or tough crust. Cornstarch contains just a trace of protein; it is mostly starch. When the cornstarch absorbs moisture the starch granules swell and become sticky, creating the bonding layer between the protein and the crumb coating mixture. Professional chefs consistently use cornstarch to dust protein which will be coated and crisp-cooked. Cornstarch works equally as well in the home kitchen. A very small amount of cornstarch, about 1/3 cup, will be sufficient for most 6-serving recipes. For most recipes I use a disposable gallon-size zip-top bag to shake protein in the cornstarch, and then tap the excess back in the bag. Discard all remaining cornstarch after use: it is contaminated with raw food. I store unused cornstarch in the refrigerator, writing the open date on the box; it should be used within six months or replaced.

Step 2: Dipping
Buttermilk: The second step in breading or crusting is to dip the dusted protein in liquid: usually eggs whisked with milk or some variation of that.

The proteins from the eggs and milk contribute to a heavier, sometimes gummy, crust. Using buttermilk eliminates the coagulation that occurs when an egg dip is used. Buttermilk produces a lighter shell that clings to the cornstarch-dusted protein. Buttermilk is the favored dipping liquid of many professional chefs. I enjoy good results using commercially available cultured buttermilk. Today's buttermilk is pasteurized, homogenized, and inoculated with lactic acid to simulate the naturally occurring bacteria in the old-fashioned buttermilk, which was the byproduct of churned butter. Another option is keeping powdered buttermilk on hand in the dry pantry. Much like powdered milk, it can be stored for many months and prepared in the precise quantity needed at the time of use. Look for it where powdered milk is sold and follow package directions for mixing.

Step 3: Coating
Crumb Mixture. The final coating in the three-step process is the crumb mixture which provides texture and flavor. Seasoned flour is traditionally used, as are bread crumbs, ground crackers, and cornmeal. Herbs and spices, ground nuts, or cheese may be added to achieve a variety of flavors. When you hear about someone's fabulous secret family recipe for fried chicken, this is the step in which the secret hides.

Dredging the wet protein works best when the crumb mixture is on a shallow pie plate or similar sided dish. The crumb mixture stays dry when using a deep-dish pie plate for the coating step. Some cooks prefer to put the crumb mixture in a bag and shake the wet protein to coat. I find this method problematic as the moisture from the dipping liquid causes the crumb coating to bind together making it ineffective for coating the remaining chicken pieces. When coating several pieces of chicken or fish it is also helpful to divide the crumb mixture, adding dry crumbs to the dredging pan as needed.

I favor panko, Japanese bread crumbs, as the foundation ingredient for the crumb mixture. The coarse crumbs make an ultra-crunchy crust receptive to an endless variety of spices, seasonings, and crusting ingredients. Panko has become so popular with home cooks it can be found in most supermarkets on the international food aisle. I generally use 2 parts panko to 1 part secondary crusting ingredient such as cracker crumbs or cornflakes. These are some of the flavor combinations I cook at my family's request.

Cornflakes and Rice Krispies®: What could be easier? Breakfast cereal is engineered to retain its crunch when in liquid. In addition, many cereals are fortified with iron and B vitamins that play a key role in our post-WLS diet and health. Avoid frosted or sugared cereals. Consider using health-wise cereals such as Special K® and protein enriched cereals such as Kashi®. **Caution:** If you are prone to "dry dipping" (eating dry cereal as a snack straight from the box, unmeasured) purchase cornflake crumbs instead of whole cereal and avoid the temptation altogether.

Roasted nuts: I originally learned about coating chicken with a crushed roasted nut mixture from TV cook Rachael Ray. Chicken coated with ground nuts stays tender and children especially love crunchy chicken nuggets made with coarse ground honey roasted nuts. **Alert!** Nut allergies are becoming more common. When cooking with nuts please tell the guests at your table which dishes contain them before the meal begins.

Parmesan: There is no resisting a Parmesan crust. Typically recipes call for 2 parts crumbs (bread crumbs, panko, cracker crumbs) to 1 part grated Parmesan cheese. The coating may be seasoned with a dry Italian herb seasoning blend, fresh or dried herbs, or simply salt and pepper. I have experimented with freshly grated Parmesan, deli-style shredded Parmigiano-Reggiano cheese, and Kraft Grated Parmesan® in the familiar green canister. Sophisticated foodies might disagree, but in my kitchen the Kraft products produce the best results when crusting protein. Shop for different grated cheeses and keep your favorite on-hand for all your crusting needs.

Whole Grain Crackers: The good news is the overabundance of quality of whole-grain crackers baked with heart-healthy monounsaturated fat and seasoned with herbs and spices. The bad news is these crackers come packaged in greater quantities than most recipes require, leaving tempting leftovers for snacking. Know your limits when it comes to potential slider foods in your pantry. One WLS cook I know uses her food processor to turn a full box of crackers into crumbs as soon as she brings them home. She stores these in an air-tight container in the freezer ready to use for crusting but unavailable and unappealing for snacking. Know your tolerance for temptation and work with it, not against it.

Soft Crackers: Saltines, butter crackers, and oyster crackers are popular soft crackers used in crusting recipes. These crackers are more porous than whole grain crackers so they will require more drizzled butter or cooking spray to achieve a nice crunch. They are best combined in equal parts with the crisper panko crumbs. In addition, soft crackers tend to lack any nutritional benefits. The inherent blandness of soft crackers is an ideal canvas for creative seasonings and crusting ingredients.

Hints for Perfect Crispy Results

Baking Powder: Baking powder is the leavening agent that produces the best results when crusting protein. Common baking powder is double acting: it will release some gas when it becomes wet and it releases more gas when exposed to oven heat. This produces tiny air pockets that contribute crispness. Do not use baking soda, it will react with the acid from the buttermilk causing the crust to rise immediately and then collapse before it goes in the oven.

Let the glue set: Once the three coating steps are complete and the protein is arranged on the prepared rack it needs to rest. Let it be for 10 to 15 minutes. On the surface it appears nothing is happening, but below the coating at the molecular level the starch is busy plumping with moisture and bonding to the protein. This waiting period is similar to letting the glue set on a craft project before moving to the next step. If the "glue" is not allowed to set properly the crust coating will likely separate from the protein and fall off during cooking, and that's just disappointing. While resting it is best to leave the protein uncovered, but if you must cover it use a clean loosely woven kitchen towel instead of plastic cling wrap.

Preheat: While the chicken rests preheat the oven to the temperature specified by the recipe. In most cases the recipe also directs the placement of the oven rack, usually the lower third of the oven. In my standard home oven that is the second level up from the bottom.

Butter drizzle: Next, prepare the fat that will be used on the crumb coating. Many recipes call for a drizzle of melted butter on the crust just before it goes in the oven. This scant amount adds to the crunch and flavor without saturating the food with oil. Another approach is to spritz the crusted pieces with butter flavored cooking spray. Try both approaches to find the one that suits you best. To add an extra dimension of flavor, drizzle garlic or herb infused olive oil in place of butter or cooking spray

Brining: If your chicken tends to be dry or if you are using boneless skinless chicken, consider soaking your chicken pieces for several hours in brine before following the steps above for crumb coating. For brine mix 4 cups of buttermilk with 4 teaspoons salt. Add chicken, cover, refrigerate for at least 1 hour and up to 8 hours. Drain and discard brine, pat chicken pieces dry. Proceed with crusting at the cornstarch step. Buttermilk brined chicken is a secret to many great fried chicken recipes. The acid in the buttermilk helps tenderize the meat and ensures that the meat retains moisture

A Note on Nutrition: Due to so many variables the nutritional values are estimated as follows: one piece of chicken provides approximately 280 calories, 26 grams protein, 9 grams fat, 3 grams carbohydrate, 0 grams dietary fiber.

Last Word - Be Prepared: Read each recipe completely and be sure to have all of the ingredients and tools in place when you begin preparation. These are not good recipes to make *"on the fly"* with missing ingredients or improper tools.

Notes:

Crispy Oven-Fried Chicken

☼ **Country Road Chef, basic oven-fried method, do not rush process**

This is the basic oven-fried chicken recipe, the platform on which you will build your soon-to-be signature dish, *"(insert name)*'s Famous Crispy Oven-Fried Chicken". I call this a Country Road Chef recipe because it does take time and thoughtfulness in the preparation. However, once you have found your own rhythm in making crispy oven-fried protein it will likely fit into the Freeway Chef category for Pace of Preparation.

Ingredients:
Protein:
12 meaty chicken pieces, bone and skin in place (breast halves, thighs, drumsticks)

Step 1: Dusting
2/3 cup cornstarch

Step 2: Dipping
2 cups buttermilk
1 teaspoon salt

Step 3: Coating
2 cups panko Japanese bread crumbs
1 cup finely crushed cornflakes
2 teaspoons poultry seasoning
1 teaspoon baking powder
1 teaspoon paprika
¼ teaspoon black pepper, freshly ground
½ cup butter

Directions: Set-up assembly line. Place cornstarch in 1-gallon zip-close bag. Mix buttermilk and salt in a deep-dish pie plate or casserole dish. In a second dish combine panko, cornflakes, poultry seasoning, baking powder, paprika, and black pepper. Prepare the tray for rack roasting: line a rimmed baking sheet with foil, shiny side up, and set a wire cooling rack on top; coat with cooking spray; set aside.

Working with a few pieces at a time, shake chicken in the cornstarch, tap to remove excess cornstarch. The cornstarch coating should be a very light dusting. Next, quickly dip each piece of chicken in the buttermilk making sure to wet it on all sides. Allow excess buttermilk to drain away. Finally, dredge in the crumb mixture, if necessary press crumbs to chicken to adhere.

Evenly space coated chicken on the prepared baking rack. Repeat the steps until all chicken pieces are coated. Discard all remaining coating ingredients, they are contaminated and should not be saved for another use.

For best results allow the chicken to rest at room temperature 10 to 15-minutes. Meanwhile, place oven rack in lower third of the oven and preheat to 375°F. While oven preheats melt butter in a small saucepan or in the microwave. Just before baking drizzle butter over chicken pieces. Bake chicken for 40 to 50 minutes, or until done. The FDA standard instructs poultry be cooked to an internal temperature of 165°F. Always test the thickest piece with an instant-read thermometer. An additional doneness test is to observe the meat juices: if chicken is sufficiently cooked the juice will run clear when meat is pierced with a fork or the tip of a knife. See the Safe Minimum Cooking Temperatures chart on page 181.

Serve Crispy Oven-Fried Chicken with any of the dipping sauce recipes on page 96. With oven-fried chicken simple fruit and vegetables are the best complex carbohydrate side dishes. Serve seasonal sliced pears, apples, or melon for a sweet side dish. For vegetable sides serve sliced tomatoes, cucumbers, carrots or a fresh green salad.

Crumb Coating Variations

Honey Roasted Peanut Crusted Chicken: Follow the method for Crispy Oven-Fried Chicken, through Step 1, Dusting, and Step 2, Dipping. Next coat the pieces in honey-pecan crusting mixture: 1 cup crushed cornflakes, ½ cup panko Japanese bread crumbs, ½ cup finely crushed honey-roasted peanuts, 1 teaspoon baking powder, 1 teaspoon paprika, ½ teaspoon pepper. Arrange on prepared baking rack and set aside. Stir 2 tablespoons honey into melted butter and drizzle chicken pieces. Bake as directed above. Serve with Honey Mustard Dipping Sauce, page 96.

Chips 'n Krispies® Oven-Fried Drumsticks: Use 8 to 10 plump chicken drumsticks. Follow the method for Crispy Oven-Fried Chicken, dusting the chicken with cornstarch and dredging in buttermilk. Coat pieces in Chips 'n Krispies crusting mixture: 2 cups crushed plain flavor potato chips, 2 cups crushed Rice Krispies®, 1 teaspoon baking powder, 1 teaspoon dried parsley, ½ teaspoon paprika, ¼ teaspoon garlic powder, ¼ teaspoon white pepper.

Arrange on prepared baking rack and set aside. Just before baking drizzle with melted butter and bake as directed above. Serve with Honey Mustard Dipping Sauce, page 96.

Maryland Oven-Fried Chicken: Follow the method for Crispy Oven-Fried Chicken, through Step 1, Dusting, and Step 2, Dipping. Next coat the pieces in crusting mixture: 2 cups crushed oyster crackers, 1 tablespoon Old Bay Seafood Seasoning, 1 teaspoon baking powder, 1 teaspoon dried parsley flakes, ½ teaspoon ground black pepper ground together in a food processor. Spritz chicken pieces with butter-flavor cooking spray and bake as directed above. Serve warm.

Honey Mustard and Onion Pretzel Crusted Chicken: Prepare the coating mixture using a food processer: place 2 cups Snyder's of Hanover® Honey Mustard Onion Pretzel Pieces in the work bowl of food processor with the chopping blade. Pulse on and off until mixture is coarsely chopped. Place pretzel crumbs in a casserole dish; with a fork stir in 1 teaspoon baking powder, 1/4 teaspoon pepper. Follow the method for Crispy Oven-Fried Chicken, through Step 1, Dusting, and Step 2, Dipping. Coat the wet chicken in the pretzel crumbs and arrange on the prepared baking rack. Just before baking spray lightly with butter-flavor cooking spray. Bake as directed above. Serve with Honey Yogurt Dipping Sauce, page 96. This coating works well on chicken nuggets or chicken tenders and garners enthusiastic praise from children.

Panko Ranch Crispy Baked Chicken: Prepare the coating mixture. Place 2 cups panko Japanese bread crumbs in casserole dish. With a fork stir in 1 (0.4 ounce) package Hidden Valley Ranch Dressing mix, 1½-teaspoons baking powder, and ½ cup grated Parmesan cheese. Follow the method for Crispy Oven-Fried Chicken, through Step 1, Dusting, and Step 2, Dipping. Coat the wet chicken in the crumb mixture and arrange on prepared baking rack. Drizzle with melted butter just before baking as directed above. Serve warm with Ranch Dipping Sauce, page 96. Hint: try this recipe with different flavored salad dressing mixes such as Italian dressing or Spicy Ranch.

Crispy Oven-Fried Coconut Chicken: Prepare the coating mixture. Mix 2 cups panko, ½ cup flaked sweetened coconut, 1 teaspoon baking powder, and ¼ teaspoon pepper in a pie plate. Using the method for Crispy Oven-Fried Chicken follow Step 1, Dusting. In Step 2 replace the buttermilk with 1 (14-ounce) can coconut milk and dip dusted chicken in it to coat. Dredge wet chicken in the panko and coconut coating pressing to adhere; arrange on prepared baking rack. Set aside to rest. Just before baking lightly spritz chicken with cooking spray. Bake as directed above. Serve warm with Honey Yogurt Dipping Sauce page 96, and sliced pineapple rings.

Cranberry and Stuffing Oven-Fried Chicken: Crush 2 cups seasoned dressing dry bread cubes; add 1 tablespoon fresh chopped parsley, place crumbs on pie plate. Pour 1 cup buttermilk, and ¼ cup cranberry sauce or cranberry jelly in another pie plate, whisk to blend. Season chicken pieces with salt and pepper; follow Oven-Fried Chicken method for step 1, Dusting; Step 2, Dipping in the cranberry buttermilk; Step 3, Coating in dressing crumb mixture: arrange on prepared baking rack. Set aside to rest. Just before baking melt ¼ cup butter and drizzle over chicken pieces. Bake as directed, serve warm with additional cranberry sauce or cranberry jelly.

Crunchy Onion Chicken: This method is similar to Quick Crunchy Chicken Tenders on page 93. Thaw 6 to 8 boneless skinless chicken breasts, pat dry. Brush both sides of chicken with reduced calorie mayonnaise. On a pie plate combine 2 cups crushed French Fried Onions and 1 cup panko bread crumbs; roll chicken in crumb coating and place on a foil lined baking sheet coated with cooking spray. Bake for 12 to 15 minutes turning once halfway through baking. Serve warm with one of the dipping sauces on page 96.

Idea Blotter: Coating Mixtures to Try

Bone-in or boneless? Skin-on or skinless? It seems there are two kinds of people: the boneless, skinless chicken eaters and the bone-in, skin-on chicken eaters. And it is not likely anyone is changing sides and I'm not going to try and convince you one way or another. I cook with both types of chicken pieces, although I prefer chicken that is cooked on the bone with the skin. To me, the chicken is more succulent and palatable. I remove the skin and don't eat it, but my husband enjoys well-seasoned crusty chicken skin. I have a negative attitude about boneless, skinless chicken breasts (the protein most Americans are likely to cook at home) because I ate my way into morbid obesity on stringy flavorless poorly made meals. That was before I learned how to prepare it with flavor and moisture.

I believe the important issue here is finding the style of chicken pieces that appeal to you. Studies show that chicken cooked with skin, but eaten with the skin removed, has no more saturated fat and cholesterol than chicken cooked without skin. Talk to your doctor or nutritionist to make an informed decision specific to your health. The chicken recipes here are versatile and most can be prepared with the type of chicken that suits you.

Food Safety - Poultry Handling: The following guidelines, provided by the FDA, reduce the risk of cross contamination and food borne illness from bacteria in that may be present in raw poultry.

No rinsing. Use poultry directly from the package, do not rinse with water. Rinsing raw poultry can cause cross-contamination in the kitchen through random splashes or run-off. Bacteria are killed by heat, not water.

Safe Zone: Prepare raw poultry away from other food. Do not allow it to come in contact with raw fruit or vegetables, canisters of ingredients, open beverages, or condiments. If available use food-safe disposable gloves when handling raw poultry and dispose of them immediately after use.

Decontaminate: Wash all tools and surfaces immediately after use with hot soapy water. If possible, wash tools and cutting boards in the dishwasher on the sterilize cycle. Use disinfecting wipes or a disinfectant solution on countertops. Wash hands with soap and warm water for 20 seconds. Dry with paper towel and dispose. Wash all cleaning rags in the hot cycle of the washing machine, adding chlorine bleach according to package directions.

Note:

Ingredients:

Directions:

Nutrition:

Chicken parmesan is one of those dishes that is universally appealing. The breaded chicken is meaty and succulent when wrapped in the crisp crumb coating flavored with Parmesan. Many recipes call for chicken *paillards* (thinly pounded chicken pieces) that cook quickly. Since the chicken is baked rather than skillet fried in this recipe I prefer to leave the breast halves in their uneven natural shape. Serve this with baked spaghetti squash or prepared spaghetti or linguini.

Ingredients:

6 (6-ounce) chicken breast halves, boneless, skinless

1/3 cup cornstarch

2 cups buttermilk

1 teaspoon salt

1 cup panko Japanese bread crumbs

1 cup crushed whole grain crackers

½ cup Kraft Grated Parmesan®

1 tablespoon dry Italian seasoning blend

1 teaspoon baking powder

½ teaspoon black pepper

½ cup butter, melted

2 – 3 cups homemade (recipe below) or prepared marinara sauce

6 ounce mozzarella cheese, grated

1 spaghetti squash, prepared as directed on page 138

SNAP!

Pictured on Front Cover

Directions: Follow the method for Crispy Oven-Fried chicken through step 1, Dusting, and Step 2, Dipping. Combine crusting ingredients (panko, crushed crackers, Parmesan, seasoning blend, baking powder, and pepper) in a pie plate and coat both sides of each chicken piece with crumbs. Arrange on prepared baking rack and set aside to rest 10 to 15 minutes. Just before baking drizzle with melted butter: bake in preheated 375°F oven for 30 to 40 minutes or until chicken is done. During the last 15 minutes of cooking place the marinara sauce in a small saucepan and heat over medium low until slightly simmering. Remove chicken from oven and lower oven temperature to 325°F. Transfer crispy chicken pieces to a baking dish in which they fit snugly, but in a single layer. Spoon ¼-cup sauce atop each chicken breast spreading to cover, leaving a border of crispy crust showing; keep remaining marinara sauce warm. Spread grated mozzarella evenly over the chicken, return to oven and bake 5 to 10 minutes for cheese to melt. Remove from oven and allow to cool slightly before serving. Place ½ cup spaghetti squash on each plate with ¼ cup warm marinara sauce and 1 piece of Parmesan chicken. Provide additional Parmesan for garnish.

Nutrition: Serves 6. Each serving provides 451 calories, 43 grams protein, 22 grams fat, 19 grams carbohydrate, 2 grams dietary fiber.

Try This: To make chicken parmesan in advance prepare the chicken pieces as directed and bake for 30 minutes in a 375°F oven. Arrange in baking dish and let them cool slightly. Cover tightly with plastic wrap and store refrigerated up to two days. One hour before serving preheat oven to 350°F. Remove from refrigerator, spoon room temperature sauce on each chicken piece and top with grated mozzarella. Cover tightly with aluminum foil, bake for 30 minutes. Remove foil and continue baking 10 minutes until cheese is melted and bubbly. Serve as directed above.

Marinara Sauce

Use this quick and easy sauce when a recipe calls for spaghetti sauce or marinara sauce. The sauce can be made 1 day in advance and refrigerated.

Ingredients:
½ cup olive oil
2 small onions, finely chopped
2 garlic cloves, finely chopped
2 stalks celery, finely chopped
2 (32-ounce) cans crushed tomatoes

Directions: In a large saucepot heat the olive oil over medium high. Add the onions and garlic and cook and stir until the onions soften, about 10 minutes. Add the celery and carrots and cook until all vegetables are soft, another 10 minutes. Add the tomatoes and simmer uncovered over low heat until the sauce thickens, stirring occasionally, about 1 hour. Adjust seasoning with salt and pepper, use as recipe directs.

☞ Indy Chef, fast and easy, multiple flavor enhancing options

This is another method for achieving a crisp coating without the three steps involved in traditional coating. A variety of protein can be prepared with this method including pork and firm fish. Children who like chicken nuggets will love these crispy chicken tenders.

Ingredients:

2/3 cup olive oil mayonnaise

2 teaspoons onion flakes

1 teaspoon dry mustard

1 cup whole grain cracker crumbs

½ cup grated Parmesan cheese

1 tablespoon parsley flakes

1 (16-ounce) package chicken tenders

> Chicken tenders are also known as chicken fingers, chicken strips, or chicken fillets. The term loosely means chicken meat without skin or bones. True chicken tenders are white meat taken from the rib meat trimmed from the chicken breast.

Directions: Preheat oven to 425°F, position rack in middle of oven. Cover a baking sheet with foil and coat with cooking spray. In a shallow bowl whisk together olive oil mayonnaise, onion flakes, and dry mustard. In a second shallow bowl combine cracker crumbs, Parmesan cheese, and parsley flakes. Working one at a time, brush mayonnaise on all sides of each chicken tender; roll in the crumb mixture to coat. Place on prepared baking sheet; repeat with all tenders. Bake for 12 to 15 minutes turning once halfway through baking. Serve warm with one of the dipping sauces on page 96.

Nutrition: Serves. Each serving provides 379 calories, 31 grams protein, 15 grams fat, 16 grams carbohydrate, trace dietary fiber.

Try This: Prepare chicken tenders as directed. Cut into bite sized pieces and arrange on top of a salad of mixed greens and fresh vegetables. Drizzle with dressing and serve for lunch. This is a good way to enjoy leftovers, if there are any. ~ Consider making a double batch, allow to cool. Arrange on a clean baking sheet and freeze 30 minutes. Package single servings and store frozen until use: reheat in microwave for a convenient meal.

Rack-Roasted Wings to Fly For

⇆Freeway Chef, one step preparation, crowd friendly, no deep-frying

When a guest declared "these wings are to die for" I had to play on those words naming them my Wings to Fly For. They are lighter that the traditional wings served at pubs and they are very good. While there is no coating step to this recipe they are baked using the rack-roasting method which produces a crisp skin and golden finish.

Ingredients:

2 tablespoons olive oil

½ teaspoon salt

½ teaspoon pepper

1 tablespoon all-purpose seasoning blend

hot sauce

16 to 20 chicken wing pieces *(wing drumettes and flat wing tips)* thawed

1 tablespoon white vinegar

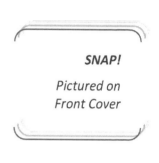

SNAP!

Pictured on Front Cover

Directions: Thaw wings if frozen. Place wings in a large bowl and drizzle with olive oil; add salt, pepper, seasoning blend, and a few dashes of hot sauce. Toss well making certain oil and seasoning is evenly distributed, let marinate at room temperature 20 to 30 minutes, tossing one more time. Ten minutes before cooking position oven rack in middle of oven and preheat to 425°F. Cover a rimmed baking sheet with aluminum foil, shiny side up, and place baking rack on top; coat with cooking spray. Douse wings with white vinegar and toss one more time; arrange on prepared baking rack and transfer to oven. Bake for 25 minutes; reduce oven temperature to 350°F and bake 10 more minutes. Serve warm, with dipping sauce of choice, page 96.

Nutrition: Each 4 wing serving provides 327 calories, 26 grams protein, 23 grams fat, 0 grams carbohydrate, 0 grams dietary fiber.

Try This: Frozen chicken wings are affordable and easy to keep on hand. Sold in large packages they are labeled ready-to-eat and include an equal portion of ice glazed first and second wing sections. Remove the amount needed for a meal counting 4 per person and thaw as directed.

A well-made dip adds moisture and flavor to vegetables, grilled protein, wraps and sandwiches. Traditional dips seem harmless enough, but they are typically high in fat and calories and we seldom eat measured portions. Early in my post-WLS life I tried to ditch the dips completely, but sometimes dry protein and crisp raw veggies need added flavor and moisture to make them palatable, particularly when we are rigorously following the liquid restrictions. Is it possible, I wondered, to make a better dip? Was there a dip that tasted good without loads of extra calories while providing protein, moisture, nutrients, vitamins, and minerals? And what about the dip-diehards around me: would they be fooled by new and improved dipping delights? Would it be possible to build a better dip with fewer calories but keep the same creamy texture and flavor of traditional ranch, onion, and other popular party dips?

So began the experimenting. Traditional ranch and onion dips are made with full-fat sour cream. I replaced the sour cream measure for measure with low-fat or no-fat yogurts. The results were too watery and failed to deliver the good feelings of satiation that come with higher-fat food. I tried setting the watery yogurt with unflavored gelatin but that was time consuming and produced inconsistent rubbery results that were not worth the trouble. Finally, I tried blending the low-fat yogurt with a small amount of full-fat mayonnaise or sour cream for the base. This achieved the result I was chasing: traditional creamy texture as the platform for all manner of flavor. Lower calories and the health benefits of low-fat dairy made this base a winner. It was indeed, a dippity-do-da-day! And the taste testers have never failed to enjoy the dip to the very last dollop.

For a creamy dip base:
¼ cup full-fat mayonnaise or sour cream
¾ cup low-fat or non-fat yogurt

Whisk with flavoring ingredients of choice until well blended. All dips should be covered and refrigerated until use. Add additional ingredients as you would when making traditional dips.

Nutrition: A traditional dip made with sour cream or mayonnaise contains 394 calories per ¼-cup serving and 47 grams fat. My light and creamy dips come in at 124 calories per ¼-cup serving and 12 grams fat. These numbers help me feel a little better with every dip.

Guacamole: In a small bowl smash one ripe peeled, pitted avocado with a fork. Fold in ¼ cup olive oil mayonnaise and ½ to ¾-cup plain low-fat yogurt. Season with salt, pepper, and hot sauce. For **Salsa-Guacamole** add ¼ to ½ cup prepared salsa to avocado mixture. Delicious with fish or chicken.

Honey Yogurt Dipping Sauce: In a small bowl combine ¾-cup plain low-fat yogurt with ¼-cup sour cream, 2 tablespoons honey; season with salt and pepper. Chill until serving. Use coarsely ground tri-colored peppercorns for interesting flavor, color, and texture.

Honey Mustard Dipping Sauce: In a small bowl whisk together ¾-cup low-fat plain Greek yogurt, ¼-cup reduced calorie mayonnaise, 1/3-cup grainy mustard, ¼-cup mild honey; season with salt. Delicious with Crispy Oven-Fried Chicken as a dipping condiment.

Ranch Dipping Sauce: In a small bowl whisk together 3/4 cup plain Greek yogurt, 1/2 cup mayonnaise, 1 (0.4-ounce) package Hidden Valley Ranch Dressing Mix, 2 green onions, whites only, minced. Cover and refrigerate 30 minutes for flavors to develop. Serve as dipping condiment with Crispy Oven-Fried Chicken and fresh raw vegetables.

Yogurt Tartar Sauce: In a small bowl place 1 cup plain low-fat yogurt, 1/4 cup olive oil mayonnaise, 2 tablespoons sweet pickle relish, 1 tablespoon lemon juice, 1 teaspoon grainy mustard, and 1/2 teaspoon dry dill. Blend well and taste for seasoning adjusting with the pickle relish, lemon juice, or mustard as needed; season with salt and pepper. Serve with crispy coated fish; store leftover sauce tightly covered and refrigerated.

Horsey Thousand Island: In a small bowl place 1 cup plain low-fat yogurt, 1/4 cup olive oil mayonnaise, ¼ cup chili sauce, 2 tablespoons pickle relish, 1 tablespoon minced onion, 1 tablespoon chopped celery, 1 teaspoon lemon juice, whisk well. Adjust seasoning with salt and pepper. Add creamy horseradish sauce 1 teaspoon at a time, taste after stirring. Continue to add a small amount of horseradish whisking and tasting, until flavor intensity is achieved. The flavor will develop slightly after the dressing is made intensifying the heat of the horseradish. This is very good with raw vegetables.

Creamy Salsa Dip: Make creamy dip base, add ¼ to ½ cup fresh salsa to base stirring to combine. Adjust flavor with salt and pepper. Serve with tacos or fajitas or as a dressing for taco salad.

Pecan Crusted Oven-Baked Chicken Kiev

⚘ Country Road Chef, inspired classic,
special occasion show-stopper

Chicken Kiev is a classic preparation where a cutlet of chicken breast is pounded and rolled around cold garlic butter and breaded, then fried or baked. The dish lost favor when mass-manufactured frozen meals were poorly made with inferior ingredients leaving a disappointing impression of Chicken Kiev. The reputation is undeserved: correctly prepared Chicken Kiev is tender, flavorful and rich. Serve it with Roasted Brussels Sprouts *(recipe follows)*. This recipe takes effort and planning resulting in a finished entree worthy of your most elegant occasion.

Ingredients:

½ cup butter, softened
1 teaspoon lemon juice
1 tablespoon fresh parsley, chopped
1 clove garlic, minced
1/4 teaspoon each salt and pepper
6 chicken breast halves, boneless, skinless
½ cup cornstarch
2 cups buttermilk
1 cup pecans, finely chopped
2/3 cup cornflake crumbs
2/3 cup bread crumbs
1 teaspoon baking powder
¼ cup butter, melted

Do not substitute margarine or non-dairy butter spread for the butter. The richness of garlic herb butter sets this dish apart from the common preparation. As with all things in health and nutrition, special occasions are to be enjoyed in moderation.

Directions: Prepare butter filling: using a wooden spoon or spatula blend butter with lemon juice, parsley, garlic, salt, and pepper. Spread mixture onto waxed paper in a 3 by 4-inch rectangle. Place in freezer to harden for 30 minutes. Meanwhile place chicken breast halves between two sheets plastic wrap; with a mallet pound to flatten to ½-inch thickness. Line a baking sheet with waxed paper; set aside. Remove butter from freezer and cut into 6 equal portions each measuring ½-inch by 4-inches. Place one portion of herb butter in center of each flattened chicken breast; fold in ends of chicken piece over butter and then fold in half and secure with toothpicks making certain butter is completely enclosed; place on prepared baking sheet. Repeat with each piece of chicken, cover with plastic wrap and refrigerate 30 minutes.

Prepare assembly line for crumb coating: place cornstarch on a plate; place buttermilk in a shallow pie plate; mix pecans, cornflakes, bread crumbs, and baking powder together on a plate. Working gently, dust chicken bundle with cornstarch, dip in buttermilk, and roll in pecan coating mixture. Return to baking sheet, and repeat until all chicken is crumb coated. Cover and refrigerate 30 minutes for crumb coating to set. About 40 minutes prior to serving position rack in middle of oven and preheat to 425°F. Coat a foil-lined baking sheet with cooking spray. Place chilled chicken bundles on baking sheet, drizzle with melted butter, and bake for 5 minutes. Without opening oven lower temperature to 400°F and bake for 25 minutes. Serve immediately: when chicken is pierced the melted butter will ooze from the chicken pooling on the dinner plate making a rich sauce for the chicken.

Nutrition: Serves 6. Each serving provides 467 calories, 38 grams protein, 29 grams fat, 11 grams carbohydrate, 1 gram dietary fiber.

Roasted Brussels Sprouts with Pecans

Prepare these delicious roasted Brussels sprouts to accompany Chicken Kiev. Use the time while chicken bundles are chilling to roast the pecans and cook the Brussels sprouts

Ingredients:

½ cup pecan halves, coarsely chopped

1 teaspoons butter

1 pound fresh Brussels sprouts, washed, trimmed

1 tablespoons olive oil

1 clove garlic, minced

1 tablespoon lemon juice

Directions: Position rack in middle of oven and preheat to 350°F. Spread pecans on rimmed baking sheet and bake until toasted and fragrant watching closely to avoid burning. Place 1 teaspoon butter in a small bowl, top with warm pecans and toss; season with salt; set aside. Coat baking sheet with cooking spray, spread Brussels sprouts evenly on tray; drizzle with olive oil, toss with minced garlic and lemon juice. Bake 25 minutes until tender, stirring once. Place in serving bowl, cover and keep warm. Just before serving toss with toasted pecans and season with salt and pepper.

Nutrition: Serves 6. Each serving provides 122 calories, 3 grams protein, 10 grams fat, 8 grams carbohydrate, 3 grams dietary fiber.

Parmesan-Sage Crusted Pork Chops

⇆Freeway Chef, juicy on the inside,
crunchy on the outside

Crusted pork prepared in the oven-fried method is succulent underneath the crunchy crust. In this recipe the traditional pork flavorings, mustard and sage, combine with Parmesan cheese for a flavorful crust.

Ingredients:

¼ cup cornstarch

1 cup buttermilk

1 tablespoon grainy mustard

1½ cup cracker crumbs

1 cup grated Parmesan cheese

1 tablespoon ground sage

1 teaspoon dry mustard

4 (4-ounce) center cut pork loin chops, trimmed of fat

Culinary sage is available in three forms: crumbled whole leaf, rubbed, and ground. Due to the intense flavor of sage the rubbed and ground forms are preferred in most preparations because a small amount will distribute evenly through the other ingredients.

1(10-ounce) jar prepared pork gravy, seasoned with 1 tablespoon grainy mustard, and ½ teaspoon sage

2 cups prepared wild rice

Directions: Line a rimmed baking sheet with foil, shiny side up, place baking rack on top, spray generously with cooking spray and set aside. Prepare assembly line placing cornstarch on one plate; combine buttermilk and grainy mustard in shallow bowl; mix cracker crumbs, Parmesan, sage, and dry mustard on plate. Working one at a time dust chops in cornstarch, dip in buttermilk mixture, coat with cracker crumbs. Arrange coated chops on baking rack making certain they are not touching. Repeat with all chops, cover loosely; set aside 15 minutes. Five minutes before cooking place oven rack in middle of oven; preheat to 375°F. Spritz coating lightly with butter flavor cooking spray, bake 15 minutes, turn, and continue baking 15 minutes longer. While the chops bake heat gravy in small saucepot whisking in mustard and sage. Serve chops warm with 1/3 cup wild rice and 1/3 cup gravy.

Nutrition: Serves 4. Each serving provides 452 calories, 26 grams protein, 16 grams fat, 52 grams carbohydrate, 3 grams dietary fiber.

Top Crusted Pork Loin Chops

⇆Freeway Chef, light crisp crust,
seared-in juicy flavor

This crusting method requires two cooking steps: searing the meat in a skillet and transferring to a baking sheet to finish in the oven. While this method means an extra pan to wash, the exceptional result is a moist piece of meat with a perfectly cooked crusty top.

Ingredients:

1 (16-ounce) pork tenderloin

¼ cup mayonnaise, reduced calorie

2 teaspoons yellow mustard

¼ teaspoon lemon pepper

¾ cup panko Japanese bread crumbs

½ teaspoon dried rubbed sage

½ teaspoon dried thyme

½ teaspoon lemon pepper

1 tablespoon olive oil

> The tenderloin comes from the full pork loin and is lean, tender, white meat pork. Pork tenderloin has a mild flavor, making it receptive to a variety of seasonings and flavors.

Directions: Cover a rimmed baking sheet with foil, shiny side up, coat with cooking spray, set aside. Preheat oven to 375°F and position rack in middle of oven. Cut pork tenderloin crosswise into four equal portions; season each piece on both sides with salt and pepper. In a small bowl mix mayonnaise, mustard, and lemon pepper. In another small bowl mix bread crumbs, sage, thyme, and lemon pepper. Heat oil in a large skillet over medium high heat; add chops and cook on each side 3 to 4 minutes; arrange on prepared baking sheet. Use a knife to spread the mayonnaise-mustard on the top of each chop. Divide crumb mixture evenly among chops, pressing into mayonnaise to adhere; spritz lightly with cooking spray. Bake for 12 to 16 minutes or until done; internal temperature should reach 145°F. Serve warm with tossed green salad or oven roasted vegetables.

Nutrition: Serves 4. Each serving provides 257 calories, 26 grams protein, 16 grams fat, 3 grams carbohydrate, 0 grams dietary fiber.

Try This: The big membership stores carry full pork loins in the fresh meat case, at a lower price per pound than packaged loin chops. Consider getting a whole loin, carving it into chops, and freezing packages with the correct number of pieces you typically prepare.

Most Americans were introduced to fish as children when we were fed fish sticks. The Gorton Company first introduced frozen ready-to-cook fish sticks in 1953 winning the Parents Magazine Seal of Approval. Minced or ground fish was formed into shapes resembling fillets or more typically long sticks, also called fish fingers. These were crusted with a batter or bread crumb coating. The home cook only had to bake the frozen fish sticks and serve to a hungry family. Ready-to-cook fish sticks continue to be popular today, although a higher grade of ready-to-cook crusted fish fillets is now available next to the minced fish preparations.

The American Heart Association recommends a well-rounded diet that includes fish as a means of preventing heart disease. Fatty fish like salmon, mackerel, herring, lake trout, sardines and albacore tuna are high in omega 3 fatty acids, the good fat credited with improving cardiovascular health.

Producing a perfectly crispy coated fish fillet from scratch is not difficult, but care must be given when cooking the fillets taking into account the density of the fish being prepared. Soft fish like tilapia or red snapper cooks very quickly; firm fish like cod or halibut takes longer to cook to doneness. Some fish is best cooked quickly in a hot skillet while others hold up to oven baking. When shopping look for fish cuts labeled "steak" for oven cooking and cuts labeled "fillet" for skillet frying.

The FDA offers basic food safety tips for buying, preparing, and storing fish and shellfish:

Purchase fresh fish that is refrigerated or displayed on ice in a covered case. Purchase frozen seafood that is sealed in the package with no sign of previous thawing. Fresh seafood should be kept cold in transport from store to home and refrigerated promptly. Frozen seafood should be placed in the freezer if it will not be used within two days. Separate fish from other foods, particularly vegetables and fruits that will be eaten raw, to avoid cross contamination. Thaw frozen seafood gradually by refrigerating overnight or placing in a sealed bag in a bowl of cold water. Cook most seafood to an internal temperature of 145°F. When serving keep cold dishes cold and hot dishes hot and leave out for no longer than 2 hours.

Cornmeal-Crusted Catfish

⇆ Freeway Chef, delicious crispy
coating, affordable and easy

For a very low caloric investment this meal provides a big value in flavor and protein. By spraying the crust with cooking spray and quickly baking in a hot oven the fish remains moist and tender wrapped in a delicious crisp crust bursting with wholesome corn flavor.

Ingredients:

2 tablespoons cornstarch

½ cup cold water

¾ cup cornflakes

¾ cup cornmeal

1 teaspoon paprika

¼ teaspoon pepper

1 teaspoon all-purpose seasoning blend, salt free

4 (4-ounce) catfish fillets fresh or frozen, thawed if frozen

Directions: In a small jar with a tight fitting lid place cornstarch and cold water. Secure top and shake vigorously until well blended and no lumps remain. Set aside. On a shallow plate mix the cornflakes, cornmeal, paprika, seasoning blend, and pepper with a fork. Line a baking sheet with foil and coat lightly with cooking spray; set aside. Working one at a time, paint both sides of each fillet with cornstarch water using a pastry brush; dip wet fillet in the cornflake crumbs; coat both sides. Place on prepared baking sheet. Follow these steps with each fillet; discard remaining cornstarch water and crumb mixture. Set pan aside to rest fillets 5 to 10 minutes *(see chicken crusting method to learn why, page 79)*. Position rack in the middle of the oven and preheat to 425°F. Spray crumb coating lightly with cooking spray; bake 8 to 10 minutes: fish is done when it flakes easily when tested with a fork. Serve warm with Yogurt Tartar Sauce, page 96.

Nutrition: Serves 4. Each serving provides 189 calories, 21 grams protein, 3 grams fat, 1 gram carbohydrate, trace dietary fiber.

Try This: This crusting recipe works well for any mild fish; try snapper, striped bass, tilapia, and flounder. ~ For fun use ground corn chips in place of the cornmeal.

Cajun-Seasoned Crispy Tilapia

Tilapia is readily available fresh or frozen. The lean flesh of tilapia is white, slightly tinged with pink, sweet and fine-textured. It's suitable for pan-frying, baking, broiling, grilling, and steaming.

Ingredients:

1 cup panko Japanese bread crumbs

½ cup cornmeal

2 teaspoons Cajun seasoning, salt-free

¼ teaspoon pepper

1 (1-pound) package tilapia fillets, fresh or frozen, thawed if frozen

1 tablespoon canola oil

1 tablespoon butter

Directions: On a shallow plate combine panko, cornmeal, Cajun seasoning, and pepper. Rinse fillets under cold running water; while still wet dredge in panko and cornmeal crumb mixture pressing to adhere crumbs to fillets. In a large, 12-inch high-sided skillet heat canola oil and butter over medium-high heat until hot. Add 3 or 4 fillets to hot skillet and cook 5 minutes on each side until fish flakes easily when tested with a fork; remove and keep warm. Repeat until all fillets are cooked. Serve warm with Yogurt Tartar Sauce, page 96, and *Quick Cajun Coleslaw*, recipe below.

Nutrition: Serves 4. Each serving provides 256 calories, 25 grams protein, 6 grams fat, 14 grams carbohydrate, 1 gram dietary fiber.

Try This: Cajun seasoning blends are widely available flavored from mild and sweet to spicy and hot. Most blends are built on a foundation of flavors that include garlic, onion, chiles, black pepper, mustard, and celery. Try several to find your favorite.

Quick Cajun Coleslaw: In a medium bowl whisk 1 cup reduced calorie ranch dressing, with 1 to 2 teaspoons Cajun seasoning blend. Add 4 green onions, chopped, and 1 (10-ounce) package ready-to-eat coleslaw salad mix. Toss together; serve chilled with Crispy Tilapia.

Cornflake-Crusted Baked Halibut

⇆ Freeway Chef, weeknight easy, special occasion feeling

Halibut is a rich meaty fish that is perfect for this crusting preparation. Serve with salad greens and sliced cucumbers for a healthy balanced meal.

Ingredients:

1 cup buttermilk

2 cups cornflake crumbs

¼ cup all-purpose flour

1 teaspoon all-purpose seasoning blend

1 teaspoon baking powder

¼ teaspoon black pepper

4 (6-ounce) halibut fillets, fresh or frozen, thawed if frozen

1 lemon, cut into wedges

> Fish is a protein source believed to be a great brain booster. Cold water fish is rich in omega 3 fatty acids, essential for brain function and development. These healthy fats have amazing brain power contributing to lowered dementia and stroke risks; slower mental decline; and they may play a vital role in enhancing memory as we age. For brain and heart health, enjoy two servings of fish each week.

Directions: Prepare assembly line: place buttermilk in a shallow bowl. On a plate mix the cornflake crumbs, flour, seasoning blend, baking powder, and black pepper. Position rack in middle of oven and preheat oven to 425°F. Cover a rimmed baking sheet with foil and coat with cooking spray. Set aside. Dip each halibut fillet in the buttermilk and then coat with crumb mixture, pressing crumbs to adhere. Place fillets on prepared baking sheet. Spritz crumb coating lightly with cooking spray. *(Note: It is not necessary to rest the fillets after coating in this recipe).* Bake 10 to 12 minutes until fish flakes easily when tested with a fork. Garnish with lemon wedges and serve warm with Yogurt Tartar Sauce, page 96.

Nutrition: Serves 4. Each serving provides 294 calories, 38 grams protein, 4 grams fat, 13 grams carbohydrate, 1 gram dietary fiber.

Try This: Prepare the Yogurt Tartar Sauce and crumb coating mixture in advance to reduce preparation time when expecting guests for this elegant entrée.

Parmesan-Crusted Baked Cod with Carrots

⇆ Freeway Chef, balanced meal,
satisfying flavors and textures

We eat with our eyes first, it is said. This dish is visually appealing as the bright carrots make a pleasing bed for the white fish crusted in pale panko and Parmesan.

Ingredients:

4 (6-ounce) cod fillets, fresh or frozen

¼ cup olive oil mayonnaise

½ cup panko Japanese bread crumbs

¼ cup Parmesan cheese, grated

1 teaspoon Old Bay Seafood Seasoning®

¼ teaspoon pepper

1 (10-ounce) package shredded carrots

1 tablespoon olive oil

1 tablespoon honey

½ teaspoon ground ginger

Cod is a saltwater fish native to the Pacific and North Atlantic Oceans. Cod's mild-flavored meat is white, lean and firm. It's available year-round and comes whole, or in large pieces. Cod can be baked, poached, braised, broiled and fried. One 3-ounce serving of cooked cod fillet provides 89 calories, 19 grams protein, 1 gram fat, no carbohydrates.

Directions: Thaw fillets, if frozen. Line a baking sheet with foil and coat with cooking spray, set aside. Position oven rack in middle of oven; preheat to 425°F. Place fillets on baking sheet and season with salt and pepper; divide mayonnaise evenly between fillets and spread to cover each. In a small bowl mix together panko, Parmesan, seasoning, and pepper; divide evenly among fillets covering each fillet completely, patting into mayonnaise. Bake uncovered for 8 to 10 minutes, test for doneness, and remove from oven or continue cooking if needed, checking after 2 to 3 minutes. The cod is done when it flakes easily with a fork. Meanwhile, in a medium skillet over high heat bring ½ cup water to boil. Add shredded carrots; reduce heat, cover, and cook 3 minutes. Uncover and cook 2 minutes longer until water evaporates. Add olive oil, honey, and ground ginger tossing well to make sure carrots are evenly coated, season with salt and pepper. Divide carrots equally among 4 plates; place fillet on carrots and serve warm.

Nutrition: Serves 4. Each serving provides 233 calories, 34 grams protein, 6 grams fat, 11 grams carbohydrate, 2 grams dietary fiber.

⇆ Freeway Chef, ridiculously healthy,
easy prep, easy clean-up

Pairing salmon with pecans is not only flavorful, it is a health-wise combination of powerful antioxidants and omega 3 fatty acids: all wrapped up in a delicious 259 calorie crispy succulent entree deserving of special occasions but easy enough for busy workdays.

Ingredients:

1 tablespoon canola oil

2 tablespoons grainy mustard

2 tablespoons honey

¼ cup panko Japanese bread crumbs

¼ cup pecans, finely chopped

1 tablespoon fresh parsley, minced

4 (4-ounce) salmon fillets, fresh or frozen, thawed if frozen

Salmon is available fresh or frozen, sold whole or cut into steaks or fillets. Salmon is also available flash frozen: look for packages with each portion individually wrapped making it easy to thaw and prepare the exact amount needed.

Directions: Position rack in middle of oven and preheat to 425°F. In a small bowl stir together canola oil, mustard, and honey. In a second small bowl mix panko, pecans, and parsley; set aside. Line a baking sheet with foil, coat with cooking spray. Place the salmon fillets on prepared baking sheet, season with salt and pepper. Brush each fillet with the honey mustard sauce; top with crumb mixture pressing lightly to adhere; spritz crumbs lightly with cooking spray. Bake for 10 to 12 minutes checking for doneness by testing with a fork. Serve warm with Honey Mustard Dipping Sauce, page 96.

Nutrition: Serves 4. Each serving provides 259 calories, 24 grams protein, 12 grams fat, 13 grams carbohydrate, 1 gram dietary fiber.

Try This: Consider making a second bowl of the honey mustard sauce to serve as a condiment with cooked fish. *(Don't use leftovers from coating the raw salmon, they are contaminated and should be discarded).* ~ Serve chilled leftover salmon on salad greens tossed with honey mustard dressing for an all new *leftover* meal.

Pecan-Crusted Trout

⇆ Freeway Chef, heart healthy, simple
ingredients and method, gourmet results

My husband and I do not fish, but we are fortunate to have many friends who fish and, more importantly, friends who share their catch. I like to return their generosity by preparing this pecan-crusted trout, taking skillet fried trout from simple to gourmet in a few simple steps.

Ingredients:

1 cup pecans

4 (6-ounce) trout fillets, with skin

juice of 1 lemon

1 cup oyster crackers

2 teaspoons dry rosemary

1 tablespoon cornstarch

½ cup cold water

2 tablespoon canola oil, divided

2 tablespoon butter, divided

lemon wedges for garnish

Directions: Toast pecan halves in a dry skillet over medium heat, shaking skillet or stirring often until pecans are crisp, and fragrant; set aside to cool. Reserve ¼ cup toasted pecans for garnish. Drizzle lemon juice on trout fillets and season with salt and pepper; set aside. Grind oyster crackers, pecans, and rosemary, in food processor; transfer to plate. In a small jar with a tight fitting lid place cornstarch and cold water; secure top and shake vigorously until well blended and no lumps remain. Brush flesh side of fillets with cornstarch wash. Press fillets flesh side down into crumb mixture, set aside and finish coating all fillets. Heat 1 tablespoon each canola oil and butter in a large skillet over medium high heat. Place two fillets, crumb side down, in skillet and cook 3 minutes. Turn with spatula and cook 3 minutes or until fish is done. Remove to plate, keep warm. Add remaining oil and butter to skillet and cook remaining two fillets as directed above. Serve warm, garnish with toasted pecans and lemon wedges.

Nutrition: Serves 4. Each serving provides 465 calories, 38 grams protein, 31 grams fat (16 grams healthy monounsaturated fat), 11 grams carbohydrate, 2 grams dietary fiber.

Baked Mahi-mahi with Macadamia Nut Crust

⇆ **Freeway Chef, crispy sweet-savory crust, attractive presentation**

This crispy heart healthy fish has a refreshing island flavor. Serve the crusted fillets with spears of fresh pineapple and small servings of sticky rice. Garnish with toasted chopped macadamia nuts.

Ingredients:

½ cup panko Japanese bread crumbs

3 tablespoons macadamia nuts, finely chopped

1 tablespoon fresh flat-leaf (Italian) parsley, finely chopped

1 cup evaporated milk

4 (5-ounce) fresh mahi-mahi fillets, about 1-inch thick

Mahi-mahi is a moderately fat fish with firm, flavorful flesh. It ranges in weight from 3 to 45 pounds and can be purchased in steaks or fillets. Mahi-mahi is best prepared simply grilled or broiled. Technically, mahi-mahi is a common dolphinfish, a surface-dwelling ray-finned fish. It is also know by the name dorado. It should not be confused with the marine mammals we adore called dolphins. The word mahi-mahi is Hawaiian for very strong.

Directions: Line a baking sheet with foil; place a wire cooling rack on the baking sheet and coat with cooking spray. Set aside. Position rack in upper-third of oven and preheat to 425°F. On a plate stir together panko, macadamia nuts, and parsley. Pour the evaporated milk in a shallow dish; dip each fillet in the milk and then dredge in the panko macadamia crumbs, pressing lightly so the mixture adheres well. Place the fillets on the rack in the baking pan making certain they do not touch. Season fillets lightly with salt and pepper. Bake in preheated oven until fish is opaque throughout when tested with the tip of a knife and the crust is golden brown, 10 to 12 minutes. Serve immediately.

Nutrition: Serves 4. Each serving provides 180 calories, 28 grams protein, 6 grams fat, 3 grams carbohydrate, 1 gram dietary fiber.

Skillet-Fried Coconut Shrimp

✿ Country Road Chef, beautiful
presentation, main dish or appetizer

Preparation early in the day makes this special occasion treat a breeze when it is time to cook and serve. For a main course dish plan three jumbo shrimp per person.

Ingredients:

¾ cup panko Japanese bread crumbs

¾ cup unsweetened shredded coconut

1 lime, zested

¼ teaspoon each salt and pepper

1 (14-ounce) can coconut milk

18 uncooked large shrimp, peeled, deveined, tails intact

¼ to ½ cup peanut oil

Directions: Early in the day at least 4 hours before cooking prepare shrimp. Line a baking sheet with waxed paper; place wire cooling rack on baking sheet; set aside. Mix together panko, shredded coconut, lime zest, and salt and pepper on a shallow plate; in a shallow bowl pour the coconut milk. Add uncooked shrimp to coconut milk and gently toss to coat. Working 1 shrimp at a time, dredge in crumb coating making sure to each shrimp is completely coated. Place on wire rack and repeat with remaining shrimp. Cover with plastic wrap and refrigerate for 4 hours allowing coating to set. Thirty-minutes before serving heat ¼ cup oil in a large deep skillet over medium high heat. Working a few shrimp at a time, fry until opaque in center and the crust turns golden, about 2 minutes per side. Transfer to paper towels to drain; continue until all shrimp are done, adding more oil as needed. Arrange shrimp on a platter and serve warm, with cocktail sauce.

Nutrition: Serves 18. One shrimp provides 120 calories, 13 grams protein, 7 grams fat, 2 grams carbohydrate, trace dietary fiber.

Cocktail Sauce: Serve shrimp with cocktail sauce *(pictured on back cover)*. Mix 1 cup bottled chili sauce with 2 teaspoons fresh lemon juice, 1 teaspoon Worcestershire sauce, 1 teaspoon hot sauce, and 1-3 teaspoons creamy horseradish sauce. Chill for 1 hour before serving with shrimp and seafood.

Note:

Ingredients:

Directions:

Nutrition:

savory sauce skillet MEALS

"It's amazing to French women how much of the same old things some people will eat. Gastronomic boredom leads to lots of unhealthy eating. If you don't make improvisation and experimentation part of your eating life, you are sure to find yourself in an eating rut. It's as bad as a romantic rut -*losing that spark*- and just as likely to get you in trouble!"
Mireille Guiliano

Sauced Skillet Meals

↪ **Indy Chef**　　⇆ **Freeway Chef**　　✩ **Country Road Chef**

Method: Skillet Chicken with Sauce

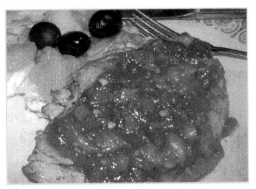

There's a cool confidence that comes when we master an essential cooking technique. It goes beyond being able to make a single recipe: it fosters the fundamental understanding of a process that empowers us to create endless dishes, all based on the method. Skillet Chicken with Sauce is a perfect example: the steps are easy, and once mastered the method yields dozens of meals that range from dinner party elegance to Indy Chef simplicity. This method and the exciting variety of flavorful sauces just may save us from tedious bland-cooked boneless skinless chicken breasts that are the demise of many well-intentioned weight management diets.

Let's begin with the basics of skillet chicken. The first goal of skillet cooked chicken is to produce a nicely caramelized, slightly crusted exterior, while keeping the inside moist and tender. The second goal is to produce a delicious pan sauce that capitalizes on the rich flavor left in the skillet after the cooked chicken is removed. Because boneless skinless chicken breasts are the most widely consumed protein in the American diet this method, and the sauce recipes that accompany it, assumes we will be using the ubiquitous ready-to-cook chicken pieces. I have developed each recipe to contain roughly 60-percent protein, 15-percent fat, and 25-percent complex carbohydrate.

Light or Dark Meat: your option. The base recipe calls for white meat boneless, skinless chicken breasts, but boneless, skinless chicken thighs are less expensive and work equally as well with the sauce variations. Personally, I prefer the darker meat chicken which is richer in flavor and tends to be moister. Dark meat chicken is higher in fat than the breast meat but the tradeoff is a higher concentration of minerals including zinc and iron. For skillet chicken bone-in pieces are not preferred because their irregular shapes, weight, and thickness make uniform cooking difficult and cooking time is extended considerably.

Skillet Chicken Basic Searing: 12 Delicious Sauces

Base Ingredients:

4 (4 to 6-ounce) boneless, skinless chicken breast halves

2 teaspoons canola oil

Sauce recipe of choice

Directions: Season chicken pieces on both sides with salt and pepper. In a large high-sided skillet, heat canola oil over medium high heat. When oil is hot add chicken pieces and sear until golden brown, about 4 minutes per side. Transfer chicken pieces to plate and tent loosely with foil to keep warm. Return skillet to heat and proceed to make the sauce of choice following the specific directions provided.

⇆ **Rosemary-Orange Chicken:** Follow the method for skillet chicken and remove seared chicken pieces to plate. Tent with foil and keep warm; return skillet to heat. Add 2 teaspoons canola oil to skillet. When oil is hot add 1 small shallot, finely chopped, and 1 clove of garlic finely chopped. Cook stirring continuously until shallot softens slightly. Add 1 cup fresh orange juice and ½ cup reduced sodium chicken broth. Bring to a simmer, cook scraping browned bits from pan, about 2 minutes. Return chicken and accumulated juices to skillet. Simmer, uncovered, until chicken is cooked through, 4 to 6 minutes. Transfer one piece of chicken to each plate. Increase heat, add 1 teaspoon butter, 1 teaspoon chopped fresh rosemary, and 1 teaspoon white wine vinegar to sauce; whisk to blend. Season the sauce with salt and pepper and spoon over chicken. Serve with a salad of sliced oranges on spinach greens dressed with citrus vinaigrette.

> These sauce variations include fruit as an ingredient. Many weight loss surgery patients who include fruit in their savory protein dishes report fewer sweet cravings following the meal. Once you perfect these sauces expand your repertoire to include a greater variety of fruits to promote healthy nutrition *and* keep your palate and eye satisfied.

⇆ **Apple Cider Chicken:** Place ¼ cup sour cream in a small bowl and set out, allowing it to warm to room temperature (see note). Follow the method for skillet chicken and remove seared chicken pieces to plate. Tent with foil and keep warm; return skillet to heat. Reduce heat to medium. Add 2 teaspoons butter to skillet. When melted add 2 peeled, cored, and thickly sliced Granny Smith apples, ¼ cup finely chopped shallot, and 1 teaspoon dried thyme. Cook and stir until apples soften, about 4 minutes. Add 1 cup apple cider; bring to a simmer. Return chicken and accumulated juices to skillet; reduce heat to low; simmer until chicken is cooked through, 4 to 6 minutes. Transfer chicken to plate and tent with foil again to keep warm. Turn off heat under skillet; add the ¼ cup room temperature sour cream and 1 tablespoon chopped fresh parsley to skillet. Stir to blend; season with salt and pepper, and spoon over chicken. *Note:* To prevent sour cream from curdling when incorporated into a hot mixture it should be at room temperature when it is added. Boiling the mixture after adding the sour cream may also cause it to curdle. While curdled sour cream is not normally a health risk it is unpleasing to look at and off-putting to some.

⇆ **Spiced Apricot Chicken:** Follow the method for skillet chicken and remove seared chicken pieces to plate. Tent with foil and keep warm; return skillet to heat. Reduce heat to medium. Add 2 teaspoons canola oil to skillet. When oil is hot add 1 small onion, chopped; 2 cloves garlic, minced; ½ teaspoon ground cumin; ¼ teaspoon ground cinnamon; and a pinch of cayenne pepper. Cook stirring, for 2 minutes. Add ½ cup unsweetened pineapple juice; ½ cup reduced sodium chicken broth; and 1/3 cup chopped dried apricots. Bring sauce to simmer, cook until slightly thickened. Return chicken and juices to skillet; reduce heat to low. Simmer until chicken is cooked through, 4 to 6 minutes. Transfer chicken to plates; season sauce with salt and pepper; spoon over chicken.

> Dark red fruits and berries contain pro-anthocyanadins – compounds that are known to support the body's vascular system. They are also powerful immunity boosters making them health-promoting complex carbohydrates to include in our high protein diet.

⇆ **Chicken with Citrus Cherry Sauce:** In a small bowl whisk together 1 cup ruby red grapefruit juice, ½ cup orange juice, and 2 teaspoons grainy mustard. Add ½ cup dried cherries; set aside. Prepare one package of instant wild rice according to package directions; keep warm. Follow the method for skillet chicken and remove seared chicken pieces to plate. Tent with foil and keep warm; return skillet to heat. Increase heat to medium high and add 1 tablespoon butter to skillet. Add juice mixture with cherries; bring to a simmer, stirring to remove browned bits from bottom of skillet. Return chicken and accumulated juices to skillet, reduce heat to a low simmer, cover and cook 10 minutes until chicken is tender and cherries are plump. Serve chicken breasts on bed of rice and drizzle with cherry sauce.

⇆ **Chicken over Rice with Plum Sauce:** Prepare 1 package instant wild rice according to package directions; set aside and keep warm. Season chicken breasts with 1 tablespoon Mrs. Dash® Extra Spicy Seasoning Blend, and follow the method for skillet chicken; remove seared chicken pieces to plate. Tent with foil and keep warm. Return skillet to heat, add 1 tablespoon olive oil and warm over medium high heat. Add 4 minced green onions, 2 cloves minced garlic, and 1 teaspoon fresh minced ginger to skillet; cook and stir 2 minutes. Stir-in 2/3-cup Chinese plum sauce (also called duck sauce) and 2 tablespoons reduced sodium soy sauce, and ¼ cup water. Whisk together and bring to a low simmer. Return chicken and accumulated juices to skillet, turning chicken breasts to coat both sides with sauce. Simmer uncovered, 6 to 8 minutes until chicken is done. Plate chicken and rice and drizzle with sauce; serve warm.

> For best results have all sauce ingredients at room temperature. This prevents cold ingredients from slowing the cooking process when added to the hot skillet.

⇆ **Chicken in Basil Cream with Sliced Tomatoes:** Follow the method for skillet chicken and remove seared chicken pieces to plate. Tent with foil and keep warm; return skillet to heat. To skillet add 1 tablespoons butter and ½ cup reduced sodium chicken broth, Bring to a simmer and scrape browned bits from bottom of skillet. Slowly stir-in 1 cup half-and-half, and 1 (4-ounce) jar sliced pimientos, drained. Simmer sauce until slightly thickened; return chicken and accumulated juices to skillet, turn pieces to completely coat in sauce. Season sauce with black pepper and top chicken with ¼ cup fresh basil leaves. Cover and simmer 6 to 8 minutes until chicken is done. Serve warm with sliced fresh tomatoes drizzled with olive oil and garnished with fresh basil sprigs.

⇆ **Chicken Breasts Provençal:** Follow the method for skillet chicken and remove seared chicken pieces to plate. Tent with foil and keep warm; return skillet to heat. Add 1 clove minced garlic, and 1 teaspoon anchovy paste to skillet and cook over medium heat, stirring, until fragrant, about 30 seconds. Add ½ cup dry white wine and bring to a boil, scraping up brown bits from bottom of skillet. Stir in 1 (14-ounce) can Italian tomatoes, ½ cup chicken broth, and 10 brine-cured black olives thinly sliced; simmer, uncovered, stirring occasionally, until mixture has thickened into a sauce, 6 to 8 minutes. Whisk in 2 tablespoons butter and accumulated chicken juices. Return chicken to skillet and simmer until done, 8 to 10 minutes. Serve chicken with sauce and garnished with fresh parsley.

⇆ **Chicken Breasts with Sun-Dried Tomato Cream Sauce:** Follow the method for skillet chicken and remove seared chicken pieces to plate. Tent with foil and keep warm; return skillet to heat. Add 1 tablespoon olive oil to skillet and warm over medium high heat. Add ½ cup coarsely chopped drained oil-packed sun-dried tomatoes, 1 small onion diced, and 2 cloves minced garlic to skillet. Cook and stir to soften vegetables; season with 1 teaspoon all-purpose seasoning blend, and salt and pepper. Add 2 cups half-and-half; 2 tablespoons tomato paste; 1 tablespoon brown sugar; cook and stir bringing up browned bits from bottom of skillet. Simmer 3 to 4 minutes allowing sauce to thicken; return chicken and accumulated juices to skillet; spoon sauce over chicken. Reduce heat to low and simmer uncovered 6 to 8 minutes until chicken is cooked and tender. Taste and adjust seasoning with salt, pepper, and all-purpose seasoning blend. Serve chicken with sauce garnished with additional chopped sun-dried tomatoes.

> Vegetables are a valuable source of nutrients and fiber and add appealing flavor and color to these easy sauces. In addition to fresh vegetables, we should include canned or frozen vegetables in our diet for a quick and balanced weeknight meal.

⇆ **Chicken with Mustard-Chive Sauce and Egg Noodles:** Prepare 2 cups (dry measure) egg noodles following package directions; keep warm. Follow the method for skillet chicken and remove seared chicken pieces to plate. Tent with foil and keep warm; return skillet to heat. Add 1 medium minced shallot to skillet and cook until softened but not browned. Reduce heat, remove skillet from heat and pour ½ cup apple brandy or Kentucky bourbon into skillet, being cautious to not let it flame. Return skillet to heat and continue cooking, allowing brandy to evaporate. Add ½ cup dry white wine to the pan; raise the heat to high, and bring it to a boil. Whisk in 3 tablespoons grainy mustard and cook allowing sauce to reduce for 1 minute. Add 1½ cups chicken broth and simmer for 2 to 3 minutes. Stir in ½-cup heavy cream and bring to a low boil. Stir in 3 tablespoons minced fresh chives. Return the chicken breasts to skillet and simmer gently until the sauce has reduced and thickened slightly, and chicken is done; about 6 minutes. To serve, put ½ cup egg noodles in the center of each plate; add 1 chicken breast and spoon ¼ cup sauce over chicken and noodles.

⇆ **Chicken with Leek and Mushroom Sauce:** Follow the method for skillet chicken and remove seared chicken pieces to plate. Tent with foil and keep warm. Return skillet to heat; add 2 teaspoons canola oil, 1 medium leek sliced, and 1 tablespoon fresh minced thyme; cook, stirring, for 2 minutes allowing leeks to wilt slightly. Add 1 (8-ounce) package sliced mushrooms; cook 5 minutes, stirring, until mushrooms and leeks are tender. Remove vegetables to plate and keep warm. Add 1 tablespoon butter and 1 tablespoon flour to skillet and whisk to blend; cook 1 minute. Slowly add 1 (14.5-ounce) can reduced sodium chicken broth to skillet; continue whisking and cooking over medium high heat until sauce is thickened. Taste and adjust seasoning with salt and pepper. Return chicken and accumulated juices to pan; smother with mushrooms and leeks. Reduce heat to low simmer, cover and continue cooking 10 minutes until chicken is done. Serve warm.

> Garlic and ginger provide more than just delicious flavor: garlic helps to protect the body from infection and ginger is an anti-inflammatory. Both add flavor and bite to skillet chicken.

⇆ **Garlic and Ginger Spiced Chicken:** Follow the method for skillet chicken and remove seared chicken pieces to plate. Tent with foil and keep warm; return skillet to heat. Add 2 teaspoons butter to skillet and melt over medium heat. Add 6 minced green onions, white and green parts, 3 cloves minced garlic, and 1 tablespoon minced fresh ginger to skillet. Cook and stir allowing vegetables to wilt and become aromatic. Add 1 cup chicken broth, 1/3 cup rice wine vinegar, 2 tablespoons of hoisin sauce, and 2 teaspoons brown sugar. Bring sauce to a simmer and cook until slightly reduced and thickened, about 3 minutes. Return chicken and accumulated juices to skillet. Reduce heat to low. Cover and simmer until chicken is cooked through, 6 to 8 minutes. Serve 1 chicken breast atop ¼ cup chow mein noodles, ¼ cup sauce, and garnished with additional minced green onions.

⇆ **Cajun Spiced Chicken with Capers and Lemon:** Season chicken breasts with 1 tablespoon Cajun-Creole seasoning mix blended with 1 teaspoon paprika and ½ teaspoon each salt and pepper. Sear chicken following the method for skillet chicken and remove to plate. Tent with foil and keep warm; return skillet to heat. Add 1 cup reduced sodium chicken broth, 2 tablespoons fresh lemon juice, and 2 tablespoons drained capers to skillet; bring to a high simmer. Cook stirring to bring browned bits from bottom of skillet; cooking until sauce thickens. Return chicken and accumulated juices to skillet; lower heat; cover and simmer 6 to 8 minutes until chicken is done. Serve warm with fresh salad greens dressed with lemon vinaigrette and garnished with lemon wedges.

Idea Blotter: Skillet Sauces to Try

Skillet Meals: A Delicious Nutritional Gift

The following recipes for skillet meals build on the basic method we learned in Skillet Chicken with Sauce. The variety here opens the possibilities of skillet cooking guaranteeing we never need be bored with the same 'ole same 'ole food again.

There is much talk and concern in the weight loss surgery community that following a metabolic surgery our bodies become malnourished because surgery impairs the normal absorption of vitamins and nutrients. Most patients are prescribed a vitamin regimen to supplement food intake in hopes of improving overall nutritional wellness. I am a big believer in taking my vitamins. But I'm also convinced that we have nothing to lose when we make certain the foods we eat provide a variety of minerals, vitamins, and nutrients. When I put recipes together it is with mindfulness to the health benefits each ingredient provides and how combining different ingredients improves the potential for absorption. What I find fascinating is the ingredients that provide powerful health benefits are the same ingredients that add a myriad of flavors and textures that take a simple skillet meal from mundane to extraordinary.

> What if my body *can* absorb all this goodness I'm feeding it? Just imagine how terrific I will feel. Preparing a meal is an opportunity to nurture a strong body, healthy heart and lungs, build immunity, and refuel our energy reserves

Occasionally one of our WLS Neighbors tells me, "My body can't absorb any nutrients, so why bother?" If it was true that our bodies cannot absorb any nutrients we would all be on medically supervised diets and dealing with feeding tubes and WLS would probably be illegal. I take a different approach asking myself, "What if my body *can* absorb all this goodness I'm feeding it? Just imagine how terrific I will feel."

When you make and enjoy these skillet meals think beyond the basic method; think about the gift you are giving your body and those who join you for a meal. Preparing a meal is not an inconvenience; an act of necessary drudgery. Preparing a meal is an opportunity to nurture a strong body, healthy heart and lungs, build immunity, and refuel our energy reserves. That makes a simple skillet dinner a pretty special gift.

You Have Arrived Skillet Chicken and Shrimp

⮀ Freeway Chef, showy presentation,
tremendous comfort food satiation

This celebratory meal is named for the LivingAfterWLS You Have Arrived motto *(page 8)*. One meal with both chicken and shrimp protein certainly isn't necessary but it is decadent and celebratory which is the aim of this dish. One serving provides two meals for me: two celebrations!

Ingredients:

1 tablespoon olive oil

4 (6-ounce) boneless skinless chicken breasts

8 medium shrimp, peeled and deveined

1 tablespoon butter

4 green onions, chopped, white and green parts

1 (10-ounce) package frozen spinach, thawed, squeezed dry

2 teaspoons all-purpose seasoning blend

¾ cup reduced sodium chicken broth

1 cup reduced fat sour cream, room temperature

SNAP!

Pictured on Front Cover

Directions: Heat olive oil in a large skillet over medium high heat. Season chicken breasts with salt and pepper, add to skillet and sear cooking on each side, about 3 to 4 minutes, until golden brown; remove to plate, tent with foil to keep warm. Add shrimp to skillet and cook 2 minutes on each side until shrimp are done and opaque in the middle; remove to plate with chicken. Add butter to skillet and melt; add green onions and cook and stir until they start to soften, add spinach, seasoning blend, and chicken broth, cooking and stirring to deglaze pan. Return chicken and accumulated juices to pan, cover and simmer 8 minutes. Stir in sour cream, turn chicken to coat all sides with creamy sauce, return shrimp to pan, cover and remove from heat, allow to stand 5 minutes. Serve 1 chicken breast, 2 shrimp and 1/3 cup sauce per person.

Nutrition: Serves 4. Each serving provides 324 calories, 47 grams protein, 12 grams fat, 6 grams carbohydrate, 2 grams dietary fiber.

Try This: Create a creamy tomato sauce by replacing the frozen spinach with 1 (15-ounce) can crushed tomatoes.

Note:

Ingredients:

Directions:

Nutrition:

Turkey Tenderloin with Mushroom Sauce

⇆ **Freeway Chef, easy turkey meal,**
creamy comforting sauce

Turkey tenderloin is 99 percent fat free turkey breast. It is available year-round in the fresh meat department so there is no thawing required. Enjoy this healthy protein in your regular menu rotation.

Ingredients:

1 (20-ounce) turkey tenderloin

2 tablespoons butter, divided

12 ounces fresh button mushrooms, sliced

1 medium sweet onion, chopped

¼ teaspoon freshly grated nutmeg

½ cup dry white wine or chicken broth, reduced sodium

1 cup evaporated milk, reduced fat

1 teaspoon cornstarch

1 tablespoon fresh chives, minced or fresh parsley, minced

Directions: Season turkey tenderloin on all sides with salt and pepper. Heat 1 tablespoon butter in a large skillet over medium high heat and cook turkey, turning to brown all sides. Continue cooking until internal temperature reaches 170°F. Remove turkey tenderloin to plate, tent with foil to keep warm. Add remaining tablespoon butter to hot skillet; add mushrooms and onions; cook and stir until tender, 5 to 6 minutes. Grate fresh nutmeg over vegetables and season with salt and pepper; add wine. Cook 2 minutes to reduce liquid, scraping any browned bits from the bottom of the skillet. In a small jar with a tight fitting lid shake the evaporated milk and cornstarch until smooth. Add to skillet and cook stirring continuously until sauce thickens. Serve sliced turkey with mushroom sauce garnished with chives or parsley.

Nutrition: Serves 4. Each serving provides 269 calories, 33 grams protein, 6 grams fat, 21 grams carbohydrate, 1 gram dietary fiber.

Try This: Add ¼ cup cranberry sauce to the mushroom sauce and capture the flavors of Thanksgiving. Serve with roasted squash or salad greens.

Turkey Scaloppini with Romaine Salad

☞Indy Chef, quick preparation, company-worthy presentation

This quick turkey scaloppini is served over salad greens making it easy to enjoy *Protein First* complimented with health promoting complex carbohydrates. The olive oil dressing contributes to nutrient absorption and lingering feelings of fullness.

Ingredients:

1 lemon

olive oil, divided

1 (6-cup) package romaine salad greens

4 green onions, sliced, white parts

1 (20-ounce) turkey tenderloin

2 tablespoons all-purpose flour

1 large tomato, diced

Directions: Wash and dry the lemon; remove zest and reserve; juice lemon into large salad bowl. Whisk in 2 teaspoons olive oil and season with salt and pepper. Add the lettuce and green onions; toss to coat; set aside. Cut turkey tenderloin into 8 equal portions. Using a meat mallet, pound each cutlet to ¼-inch thickness. Season cutlets with salt, pepper, and lemon zest; lightly dust each side with flour. In a large skillet heat 1 tablespoon olive oil over medium high heat. Working a few at a time cook cutlets for 2 to 4 minutes per side until golden brown and cooked through: remove to plate and keep warm. Deglaze skillet with ½ cup chicken broth and 1 tablespoon lemon juice. Serve 2 cutlets per person drizzled with pan sauce and accompanied with romaine salad and diced tomato.

> Turkey breast is the leanest of all meats. It has a mild flavor that makes it receptive to a host of different flavors and preparations. There are 26 grams lean protein in a 3-ounce serving that also provides goodly amounts of niacin and vitamin B6. Lean turkey breast is sold as tenderloin, cutlets, ground turkey, and turkey sausage.

Nutrition: Serves 4. Each serving provides 216 calories, 30 grams protein, 7 grams fat, 8 grams carbohydrate, 2 grams dietary fiber.

Try This: Add freshly grated Parmesan cheese and croutons to the salad greens for Turkey Scaloppini Caeser salad.

Sweet Italian Turkey Sausage with Veggies and Pasta

⇆ Freeway Chef, colorful variety,
succulent sausage flavor

This is a good recipe for learning to enjoy pasta as an ingredient in our meal rather than the main course. The sausage and vegetables play the lead role providing most of the volume while pasta makes an appearance as supporting cast. Learn more about including pasta in your *Protein First* diet on Page 165.

Ingredients:

1½-cup garden rotini corkscrew pasta
1 (19-ounce) package Jennie-O® Lean Sweet Italian Turkey Sausage
2 tablespoons canola oil
1 medium red onion, thinly sliced
1 yellow sweet bell pepper, seeded, chopped
2 cloves garlic, minced
2 green zucchini, halved lengthwise, cut into 1/2-inch pieces
1 pint cherry tomatoes, rinsed and drained
1 cup barbecue sauce, any flavor

Directions: Cook pasta according to package directions, drain and set aside. Slice sausage links into 1-inch pieces; set aside. Prepare all vegetables. In large high-sided skillet heat canola oil over high heat; add turkey sausage and cook and stir until sausage is lightly browned and fragrant. Add onion, bell pepper, garlic, and zucchini. Continue to cook and stir over high heat until vegetables become tender but not overly soft. Add cherry tomatoes and cooked pasta and cook another 2 minutes. Stir in barbecue sauce and ½ cup water; toss to coat all vegetables and sausage; adjust with more barbecue sauce or water to preferred consistency. Serve warm.

Nutrition: Serves 4 to 6. Each 2-cup serving provides 322 calories, 21 grams protein, 9 grams fat, 44 grams carbohydrate, 8 grams dietary fiber.

Try This: Vary the vegetables with the season and use frozen vegetable blends when fresh vegetables are in short supply. ~ Chilled leftovers of this skillet meal make an easy on-the-go lunch. Serve leftovers chilled, or gently reheated in the microwave.

Black Bean Turkey Tacos

Tacos are notoriously high in fat. This take on tacos lowers the fat while flavor is boosted by salsa and black beans mixed with ground turkey. A quick meal with all the taco trimmings we love: it's time for taco night!

Ingredients:

1 tablespoon canola oil

1 (20-ounce) package ground turkey

1 tablespoon taco seasoning

1 (15-ounce) can black beans, rinsed and drained

1 clove garlic, minced

½ cup salsa

2 tablespoons ketchup

1 large tomato, diced

1 package shredded lettuce

1 bunch green onions, sliced

1 (8-ounce) package Cheddar, shredded

Suggested toppings: taco sauce, sour cream, salsa, and guacamole.

8 (8-inch) tortillas or taco shells

> The nutrients in black beans provide steady energy from the B vitamin group. Unlike the energy that comes from simple sugars *–energy boosts that surge and fizzle out--* steady energy fuels the body consistently over longer periods of time without highs and lows.

Directions: Heat canola oil in a large skillet over medium high heat; crumble ground turkey into skillet; add taco seasoning blend. Cook and stir until turkey is done; add black beans, minced garlic, ½-cup salsa, and ketchup. Lower heat and simmer until sauce is reduced and flavors blended. Meanwhile prepare taco topping tray by arranging tomato, lettuce, green onions, and shredded Cheddar on a serving platter. Place sour cream, salsa, and guacamole in small bowls with spoons for serving. Warm tortillas following the package directions. Place turkey and black bean filling in a serving bowl. Serve buffet style, everyone preparing their own taco masterpiece

Nutrition: Makes 8 tacos. Each taco provides 280 calories, 24 grams protein, 2 grams fat, 11 grams carbohydrate, 3 grams dietary fiber. *(Nutrition will vary with toppings).*

Beef Tenders with Horseradish Sauce

⮌Freeway chef, easy preparation,
affordable cut of beef

Beef and horseradish are a classic pairing. The sauce here, made with Greek yogurt, provides just the right balance of creamy coolness and spicy kick. Mashed Garlic Cauliflower is a low-carb, low-glycemic alternative to mashed potatoes. The flavor is similar to mashed potatoes and they make a neutral compliment to the pungently spicy flavor of the horseradish sauce.

Ingredients:

1 (20-ounce) beef sirloin tip steak

1 teaspoon all-purpose seasoning blend

1 tablespoon canola oil

1½ cup beef broth, low sodium

1 cup Greek yogurt, plain, reduced fat

2 tablespoons prepared creamy horseradish

Mashed Garlic Cauliflower

Directions: To make slicing easier freeze beef sirloin 5 to 10 minutes; slice against the grain into ¼-inch thick strips. Season steak strips with salt, pepper, and seasoning blend. In a large skillet heat canola oil over medium high heat; add beef. Cook and stir until beef is browned on all sides and cooked. Deglaze pan with beef broth and simmer until broth is reduced, about 6 minutes. In a small bowl whisk together Greek yogurt and horseradish until combined. Stir ¼ cup into steak, coating all pieces; serve beef with remaining horseradish yogurt and *Mashed Garlic Cauliflower*.

Nutrition: Serves 4. Each serving provides 243 calories, 32 grams protein, 11 grams fat, 2 grams carbohydrate, 0 grams dietary fiber.

Mashed Garlic Cauliflower: In a steamer basket or microwave cook 8 cups cauliflower florets until very tender. Allow to cool slightly. Place cauliflower in bowl of food processor with 2 cloves garlic. Add 1/3 cup Greek yogurt, 2 teaspoons olive oil, 1 teaspoon butter; season with salt and pepper. Pulse several times until cauliflower is smooth and creamy; add more yogurt if necessary to reach preferred consistency. Place mashed cauliflower in microwave safe serving bowl and heat until steaming; serve warm. **Nutrition:** Each ¾-cup serving provides: 107 calories, 5 grams protein, 7 grams fat, 12 grams carbohydrate, 5 grams dietary fiber.

Beef and Broccoli Stir-Fry

☞ Indy Chef, fast cooking, healthy balance of protein and vegetables

Prepare all ingredients before beginning to cook. Traditional stir fry cooking is very fast requiring constant stirring from start to finish.

Ingredients:

cornstarch

½ teaspoon garlic powder

1 (16-ounce) beef sirloin steak, trimmed, cut into thin strips

canola oil

4 cups broccoli florets

1 small onion, cut into wedges

1 clove garlic, minced

1 teaspoon fresh ginger, minced

4 ounces button mushrooms, sliced

1/3 cup soy sauce, reduced sodium

2 tablespoons brown sugar

1 teaspoon ground ginger

1 (5-ounce) can chow mein noodles

> A wok is a round-bottomed cooking vessel popular in Asian cooking, where its uses include stir-frying and steaming. Woks are fairly common in American households, particularly electric woks. Most are made with non-stick coating so little cooking fat is needed to keep the vegetables and protein from sticking in the fast-paced cooking method.

Directions: In a large non-reactive bowl whisk together 2 tablespoons cornstarch, garlic powder, and ¼ cup of cold water. Add sirloin strips and toss to coat; set aside. In a small bowl combine soy sauce, brown sugar, ground ginger, 1 tablespoon cornstarch, and 2 tablespoons of water, whisking to blend; set aside. In a large skillet or wok heat 1 tablespoon canola oil until very hot; add beef and cook, stirring continuously, until beef is cooked. Remove beef to plate, tent with foil. Add 1 tablespoon canola oil to hot skillet or wok; add broccoli, onions, garlic, ginger, and mushrooms; cooking and tossing until crisp-tender. Add cooked beef and accumulated juices to vegetables; add soy sauce mixture; cook and stir for 2 minutes until sauce is thick and coats vegetables and beef. Serve immediately; divide beef and broccoli evenly among four plates; top each serving with ½ cup chow mein noodles.

Nutrition: Serves 4. Each serving provides 401 calories, 30 grams protein, 19 grams fat, 28 grams carbohydrate, 4 grams dietary fiber.

⌔ **Indy Chef, satisfies carb cravings,
beef provides potent protein nutrients**

This is a complete meal with the perfect balance of protein, complex carbohydrate, dietary fat, and whole grain carbohydrates found in the heart-healthy soba noodles.

Ingredients:

1 (8-ounce) package whole grain soba noodles
¼ cup hoisin sauce
3 tablespoons soy sauce, reduced sodium
1 teaspoon five-spice powder
1 (16-ounce) flank steak, trimmed, cut into ¼-inch strips
2 teaspoons canola oil
2 green onions, minced
2 teaspoons bottled minced garlic
2 ripe tomatoes, each cut into 6 wedges
2 green onions; cut into ½-inch pieces
1 tablespoon fresh basil, chopped

Chinese five-spice powder is a pungent mixture of five ground spices. Most five-spice blends combine equal parts of cinnamon, cloves, fennel seed, star anise, and Szechuan peppercorns. Look for it on the spice aisle of your favorite grocery store.

Directions: Cook soba noodles according to package directions. While noodles cook, combine hoisin sauce, soy sauce, five-spice powder, and steak in a large bowl; toss to coat. In a large high-sided skillet or wok heat oil over high heat. Add minced green onions and garlic; cook and stir 30 seconds until aromatic. Add beef mixture; cook 5 minutes stirring frequently. Add tomato wedges and green onion pieces; cook 2 minutes. Divide soba noodles among four plates and top each with equal portions of the beef mixture.

Nutrition: Serves 4. Each serving provides 374 calories, 28 grams protein, 12 grams fat, 36 grams carbohydrate, 2 grams dietary fiber.

Try This: This recipe adapts easily to different protein. Try it with poultry, firm fish, or shellfish. ~ Add red or yellow bell peppers to include more antioxidant immunity boosting nutrients in your diet. ~ Hoisin sauce provides sweet and spicy complex flavor. Find bottled Hoisin sauce, also called Peking sauce, on the International foods aisle.

℘ **Indy Chef, colorful presentation,**
smoky chipotle flavor

The fajita is relatively new to the American food scene having gained popularity in the 1990s. The dish originated in the cattle camps of southwest Texas in the 1930s when Mexican vaqueros (cowboys) used skirt steak to make a fast meal of spicy meat and peppers wrapped in tortillas.

Ingredients:

1 (24-ounce) skirt steak, thinly sliced against the grain
1 tablespoon Mrs. Dash® Southwest Chipotle Seasoning Blend, salt-free
2 tablespoon canola oil
1 red bell pepper, seeded, sliced lengthwise
1 green bell pepper, seeded, sliced lengthwise
1 small onion, thinly sliced
1 tablespoon soy sauce, reduced sodium
1 tablespoon brown sugar
1 tablespoon chipotle canned in adobo sauce
8 (8-inch) flour fajita tortillas
Toppings: 1 avocado, sliced; ½ cup sour cream

Directions: Place sliced steak in a large bowl, sprinkle with seasoning blend and toss to coat; set aside. In a large skillet heat 1 tablespoon canola oil over high heat; add red and green bell pepper, and onion. Cook and stir vegetables over high heat cooking them rapidly until tender, about 5 minutes. Remove to plate; tent with foil to keep warm. Add remaining canola oil to skillet and heat until smoking; add steak and cook quickly, stirring until steak is browned on all sides. Add the soy sauce, brown sugar, and canned chipotle; stir to combine. Toss in cooked peppers and onion; remove from heat, cover and keep hot. Warm the tortillas according to package directions. Serve family style with avocado and sour cream for toppings.

Nutrition: Makes 8 fajitas. Each fajita provides 422 calories, 23 grams protein, 16 grams fat, 45 grams carbohydrate, 3 grams dietary fiber.

Try This: Use leftovers for lunch. Store tortillas separate from meat and pepper filling; heat separately in microwave and assemble for a warm midday meal. ~ For convenience purchase bottled fajita sauce and follow label directions.

A few words on pork

In May 2011 the United States Department of Agriculture announced new cooking guidelines for pork and this is great news for weight loss surgery patients. The old guidelines called for cooking pork to an internal temperature of 160°F. These high cooking temperatures were appropriate many years ago when pork contained much more fat and was also prone to carrying food borne illness. Advances in pork breeding now produce a leaner meat and improved standards in farming have decreased the chance of pork carrying illness causing bacteria.

Now we may safely cook pork to an internal temperature of 145°F. Cooked to this standard pork is juicier and more palatable. For those of us with weight loss surgery and following the liquid restrictions *(no liquid with meals)* a more succulent piece of meat is essential for our culinary enjoyment and pouch comfort.

Both the USDA and the National Pork Board recommend using a digital instant-read thermometer to ensure an accurate final cooked temperature. Ground pork, like all ground meat, should be cooked to 160°F. Pre-cooked ham can be reheated to 140°F, or enjoyed cold on sandwiches.

Supporting weight loss: According to a study published in the February 2011 Journal of Obesity, Purdue University researchers found that including protein from lean pork in your diet can help you lose weight while maintaining more lean tissue, including muscle. Dieters eating pork rated themselves more positively in terms of overall mood and feelings of pleasure during dieting compared to those who ate less protein from other sources. The participants in the study followed either a high protein diet or a normal protein diet of the same amount of calories. The participants who ate more protein, with pork as their only source of meat, felt fuller longer after meals.

Pork truly is The Other White Meat® According to recent analysis by the US Department of Agriculture pork tenderloin contains the same amount of fat and slightly fewer calories than the same size serving of skinless chicken breast. What's more, the USDA found there are several cuts of pork that are considered either extra lean or lean by labeling standards. This lower fat pork adds to the variety of meat we can enjoy when following our high protein diet. Look for pork labeled "Lean" or "Extra Lean" to enjoy the lean protein benefits in a WLS diet.

Pork Chops with Lemon-Mustard Sauce

⇆ Freeway Chef, aromatic appeal,
tangy fresh flavors, moist and meaty

Avoid overcooking pork which will leave it dry, tough, and unappetizing. Use an instant-read meat thermometer inserted horizontally to measure doneness. Cook to 145°F and remove from heat; allow to stand off the heat for 5 minutes so the proteins relax and plump with juice, making a moist, delicious, properly cooked chop.

Ingredients:

4 (6-ounce) pork loin chops, 1-inch thick, boneless

1 tablespoon canola oil

½ cup chicken broth, reduced sodium

1 lemon, zest removed and reserved, juiced

2 tablespoons grainy mustard

1 clove garlic, minced

½ teaspoon dried rosemary, crushed

1 lemon, cut into wedges

Directions: Season pork chops on both sides with salt and pepper; set aside. In a large skillet, heat canola oil over medium high heat. Place pork chops in skillet making sure they do not touch; cook 4 to 6 minutes, turn, cook additional 4 to 6 minutes until done. Internal temperature should measure 145°F. Remove chops to plate, tent with foil and keep warm. Lower heat to medium and add chicken broth to skillet. Cook and stir scraping browned bits from pan; add 2 tablespoons lemon juice, mustard, garlic, and rosemary. Cook sauce on low simmer until reduced, about 5 minutes. Serve each pork chop topped with 2 tablespoons lemon-mustard sauce and garnished with lemon zest and lemon wedge.

Nutrition: Serves 4. Each serving provides 260 calories, 39 grams protein, 10 grams fat, 1 gram carbohydrate, trace dietary fiber.

Try This: Buttered green beans with a squeeze of fresh lemon juice are a perfect vegetable carbohydrate to complement these chops. ~ Serve leftover pork thinly sliced on salad greens topped with honey mustard dressing.

Pork Chops with Onions and Apples

⇆ Freeway Chef, autumnal aromas and flavors, superior skillet meal

Pork chops with apples always signal the arrival of autumn for me. I love the complementary flavors of pork and apple as they meld together in a perfect meal of sweet and savory goodness.

Ingredients:

2 teaspoons freshly ground black pepper

2 teaspoon kosher salt

½ teaspoon garlic powder

4 (6-ounce) pork loin chops, 1-inch thick

1 tablespoon canola oil

2 medium onions, sliced into rings

2 medium tart apples, cored, sliced

1 tablespoon lemon juice

2 tablespoons brown sugar

½ teaspoon ground cinnamon

2 tablespoon butter

> Apples stimulate the growth of beneficial bacteria in the digestive tract. They also contain pectin, which helps remove excess cholesterol and toxic metals.

Directions: In a small bowl combine black pepper, salt, and garlic powder; rub seasoning on both sides of each pork chop. In a large high-sided skillet heat canola oil over medium high heat. Add seasoned pork chops and cook 4 to 6 minutes per side. Meanwhile, in a medium bowl toss apples and onions with lemon juice, brown sugar, and ground cinnamon. Once pork chops are browned on both sides and nearly cooked, remove to plate and tent with foil to keep warm. Melt butter in skillet and scrape browned bits from bottom of pan. Add seasoned apples and onions and cook 4 to 5 minutes to soften. Return pork chops to skillet nestling them among apples and onions. Reduce heat to medium low, cover, cook for 8 to 10 minutes. Serve warm with one chop and ½ cup apples and onions per serving.

Nutrition: Serves 4. Each serving provides 371 calories, 38 grams protein, 16 grams fat, 19 grams carbohydrate, 2 grams dietary fiber.

Try This: If apple mixture seems dry, which may happen depending on moisture content in apples, add ¼ to ½-cup water or apple juice. The pan sauce is truly the "icing on the cake" in this recipe: Enjoy it! ~ For extra cinnamon flavor and aroma add a 4-inch cinnamon stick with the apples; remove and discard before serving.

Pork Medallions with Creamy Double Apple Sauce

⇆ Freeway Chef, creamy satiating
sauce, effortless elegance

This is a different take on pork chops and apples; the creamy sauce flavored with apple cider is intensely comforting. Add steamed butternut squash for a full-course, beautiful, and healthy meal.

Ingredients:

2 cups wide egg noodles, uncooked

2 cups apple cider, divided

2 large tart green apples, peeled and cut into 8 wedges each

1 (16-ounce) pork tenderloin, trimmed, cut into ½-inch thick slices

½ teaspoon dried rosemary, crushed

1 tablespoon olive oil

½ cup half-and-half

fresh parsley sprigs for garnish

Directions: Prepare egg noodles following package directions, adding 1 cup apple cider to cooking water. While noodles cook bring remaining 1 cup apple cider to boil in a large high-sided skillet. Add apple wedges; reduce heat and simmer 5 minutes or until apples begin to soften. Remove apples with a slotted spoon and place in a medium bowl. Continue to cook cider until reduced; pour reduced cider over apples; set aside. Season pork chops with salt, pepper, and dried rosemary. Add olive oil to skillet over medium high heat. Sear pork chops, cooking about 4 minutes per side, until browned and cooked through. Return apples to skillet and stir-in half-and-half; bring to a low simmer. Serve two chops over ½ cup egg noodles, topped with 4 apple wedges and ¼ cup of sauce, garnished with parsley sprigs.

Nutrition: Serves 4. Each serving provides 345 calories, 29 grams protein, 12 grams fat, 28 grams carbohydrate, 2 grams dietary fiber.

Try This: To cook pork more quickly slice against the grain in thin strips and cook and stir in olive oil over medium high heat. Slicing the pork into strips rather than medallions will help stretch the recipe to feed more people should you find yourself making room for unexpected guests at your table.

Garlic-Pepper Pork Chops with Peach-Vinegar Glaze

⇆ Freeway Chef, sweet and savory, terrific use of fresh ripe peaches

This is one of my favorite pork recipes because it is beautiful to prepare, wonderfully flavored, and totally unpredictable. We all expect apples to be paired with pork. But peaches and hot peppers with pork is new and tantalizing and the results are gourmet spectacular for a Freeway Chef meal. Don't save this for a special occasion; treat yourself tonight.

Ingredients:

4 (6-ounce) boneless pork chops

1 teaspoon garlic pepper seasoning blend

2 teaspoons olive oil

½ small red onion, chopped

1 jalapeño chile, seeded and minced

1 cup chicken broth

½ cup peach jam

2 tablespoons balsamic vinegar

4 ripe peaches, peeled and quartered

1 bunch fresh cilantro or parsley, chopped

Peaches compliment pork beautifully, and they are a good fruit to include in the WLS diet. At only 37 calories one medium peach provides 10 grams complex carbohydrate and 2 grams dietary fiber. They rank low on the Glycemic Index so when eating them with pork blood sugar levels will hold steady.

Directions: Rub chops on both sides with garlic pepper seasoning. Heat olive oil in a large skillet over medium-high heat and cook chops to brown on one side; turn chops; add onion and jalapeño chile to pan. Continue to cook, stirring occasionally, until onion is tender, 2 to 4 minutes. Add chicken broth, peach jam and vinegar; cover, lower heat and simmer 8 to 10 minutes. Serve chops with pan sauce and peach quarters; garnish with cilantro or parsley.

Nutrition: Serves 4. Each serving provides 334 calories, 44 grams protein, 18 grams fat, 32 grams carbohydrate, 4 grams dietary fiber.

Try This: Use pears or plums in place of the peaches matching pear or plum jam appropriately. Pork goes well with many stone fruits; cooking with a variety of fresh fruit keeps the menu interesting and adds nutrients, vitamins, and dietary fiber to meals. ~ During the off-season use fruit canned in natural juices with no added sugar in place of fresh.

Skillet Salmon with Mushroom-Shallot Sauce

⏩Indy Chef, one pan meal, high protein; heart healthy omega 3 fats

This recipe is easy to adjust for the number of people who are eating. Simply cook one fillet per person. Leftover salmon is terrific tossed with greens and vinaigrette for a second meal later in the week.

Ingredients:

2 teaspoons olive oil

4 (4-ounce) fresh or frozen skinless salmon fillets, thawed if frozen

1 (8-ounce) package button mushrooms, sliced

1 medium shallot, finely chopped

½ cup dry white wine or reduced sodium chicken broth

1 tablespoon Dijon-style mustard

2 teaspoons fresh thyme, snipped

Directions: Warm olive oil in a large skillet over medium heat. Season salmon fillets with salt and pepper; add to skillet and cook 4 to 6 minutes on each side until done and fish flakes easily. Remove from skillet to plate; tent with foil to keep warm. Add mushrooms and shallot to skillet and cook and stir over medium high until mushrooms are tender and shallots are fragrant. Add wine, mustard, and thyme; continue cooking, stirring to pull browned bits from bottom of skillet. Serve 1 salmon fillet topped with mushrooms and sauce.

Nutrition: Serves 4. Each serving provides 285 calories, 24 grams protein, 18 grams fat, 2 grams carbohydrate, trace dietary fiber.

Learning: Shallots are a member of the onion family but they are formed more like garlic than onions, with a head composed of multiple cloves, each covered with a thin, papery skin. The skin color can vary from pale brown to pale gray to rose, and the off-white flesh is usually tinged with green or purple. Shallots are favored for their mild onion flavor and can be used in the same manner as onions. Choose dry-skinned shallots that are plump and firm; there should be no sign of wrinkling or sprouting. Store dry shallots in a cool, dry, well-ventilated place for up to a month.

Pineapple Glazed White Fish with Broccoli

☞ Indy Chef, no-prep ingredients, nutritionally balanced and delicious

This meal is perfect for nights when there is no time for chopping or preparing ingredients. The sauce is uncomplicated and works well to marry the flavor of the fish with the steamed broccoli.

Ingredients:

1 (8-ounce) can unsweetened sliced pineapple

1½ teaspoons cornstarch

¼ teaspoon ground ginger

2 tablespoons honey

2 tablespoons soy sauce

1 tablespoon lemon juice

1 (16-ounce) package broccoli florets, ready-to-eat

4 (6-ounce) fillets white fish (tilapia, cod, sole, flounder)

> Pineapple is a tropical fruit loaded with enzymes that can aid digestion and reduce inflammation. Include fresh and canned pineapple in your healthy weight management diet.

Directions: Drain and reserve pineapple juice, set aside. In a small saucepan over medium heat combine cornstarch and ginger; add reserved pineapple juice whisking to combine. Add honey, soy sauce, and lemon juice; bring to a boil. Cook and stir until sauce thickens, 1 to 2 minutes. Set aside. Place broccoli florets in a microwave safe container, add 2 tablespoons water, cover with plastic wrap and microwave on high 4 to 6 minutes until crisp-tender. Drain liquid, season with salt and pepper, toss with 2 tablespoons pineapple glaze; set aside. Coat a large skillet with cooking spray and place over medium high heat. When skillet is hot, add fish fillets; cook uncovered 4 minutes; turn fillets and continue cooking until done and fish flakes easily when tested with a fork. While second side of fillets cooks spoon sauce over fillets; top with 1 or 2 pineapple rings. Remove from heat, cover and let stand 5 minutes. Serve warm with pineapple glazed broccoli.

Nutrition: Serves 4. Each serving provides 248 calories, 36 grams protein, 2 grams fat, 21 grams carbohydrate, 4 grams dietary fiber

Try This: This recipe lends itself to most mild fish and the glaze nicely compliments most lightly steamed vegetables.

Shrimp Fra Diavolo

⇆ Freeway Chef, seafood house entrée,
pantry ingredients for quick fixing

Fra Diavolo is the classic designation for an Italian-American dish in which protein is drenched in spicy tomato sauce. By using a prepared commercial or homemade marinara sauce this recipe comes together quickly.

Ingredients:

1 (16-ounce) package angel hair pasta
1½ pounds medium to large shrimp, peeled, deveined, uncooked
1 tablespoon olive oil
1 tablespoons butter
2 cloves garlic, finely chopped
¼ to 1 teaspoon crushed red pepper flakes
1 (26 to 32-ounce) jar prepared commercial or homemade marinara sauce
1 bunch fresh parsley

Directions: Prepare angel hair pasta according to package directions; drain, and keep warm. Rinse shrimp; drain in colander, pat dry. Place a large skillet on medium high heat; add olive oil and butter; heat until butter melts and combines with olive oil. Add shrimp; cook on each side 3 to 4 minutes until pink and opaque in the middle. Using a slotted spoon, remove the shrimp to plate; tent with foil to keep warm. Add garlic and red pepper flakes to cooking liquid; cook and stir until fragrant, about 3 minutes. Add prepared marinara sauce and cook and stir until bubbling. Remove from heat; toss shrimp with sauce. Place 1/3 cup angel hair pasta on each plate and top with 1 cup of shrimp and sauce. Garnish with parsley. To lower calories replace pasta with steamed spaghetti squash.

Nutrition: Serves 6. Each serving provides 476 calories, 30 grams protein, 9 grams fat, 67 grams carbohydrate, 4 grams dietary fiber.

Steamed Spaghetti Squash: Pierce 1 (3 to 4 pound) spaghetti squash with a small sharp knife to prevent bursting. Microwave on high 6 to 8 minutes; turn and cook 6 to 8 minutes more until squash feels slightly soft; cool 10 minutes. Carefully open squash lengthwise; remove and discard seeds. Scrape squash flesh into bowl with a fork, loosening and separating strands. **Nutrition:** 1 serving ½ cup spaghetti squash, 1 cup shrimp and sauce: 211 calories, 21 grams protein, 8 grams fat, 14 grams carbohydrate, 2 grams dietary fiber.

Halibut with Green Onions and Summer Squash

⇆Freeway Chef, simple ingredients, sophisticated flavors and presentation

Halibut is classed as a meaty fish and considered a valuable source of high quality lean protein. In addition to protein, halibut provides B vitamins, potassium, and iodine: minerals that support proper thyroid function.

Ingredients:

8 green onions, bulbs separated from tops

olive oil, divided

1½ pounds assorted summer squash, cut into 1-inch pieces

1 tablespoon thyme leaves plus 4 sprigs fresh thyme

4 (6-ounce) skinless fresh or frozen halibut fillets, thawed if frozen

1 lemon, cut into wedges

> When you need to add more cooking oil to a hot skillet with ingredients already cooking, tilt the skillet moving food to one side. Center the empty side over heat; add oil allowing time to raise oil temperature before mixing with other ingredients.

Directions: Cut green onion bulbs in half lengthwise (quarter if large). Cut enough green onion tops into 1-inch lengths to measure 1 cup; set aside. Heat 1 tablespoon olive oil in a large skillet over medium high heat until almost smoking; add onion bulbs, cut side down; cook until golden, about 3 minutes. Transfer to a plate. Add 1 tablespoon olive oil to skillet; add squash; cook and stir until golden and just tender, about 5 minutes. Stir in onion bulbs, 1 cup onion tops, and 1 tablespoon thyme leaves. Season with salt and pepper and cook until green onion tops wilt, about 2 minutes. Place vegetables in a bowl and loosely cover with foil to keep warm. Return skillet to medium high heat, add 2 tablespoons olive oil. Season halibut fillets with salt and pepper; add to skillet and cook 3 to 4 minutes per side until cooked through and opaque in center. Divide onion and squash among four plates and top each with one halibut fillet, a sprig of thyme and lemon wedge.

Nutrition: Serves 4. Each serving provides 348 calories, 38 grams protein, 18 grams fat, 9 grams carbohydrate, 4 grams dietary fiber.

Try This: This vegetable sauté is a good opportunity to add fresh seasonal vegetables to a meal. Add cherry tomatoes, eggplant, green beans, squash, mushrooms, or anything to make the dish uniquely yours.

Note:

Ingredients:

Directions:

Nutrition:

OVEN *Baking*
ROASTING
moist braising
and slow cooker meals

> *"There is no more giddy smell for a meat eater than a good piece of beef roasting in the oven."*
> Barbara Kafka

Oven Baking, Roasting, Moist Braising and Slow Cooking

Methods and Articles:

Recipes:

↫ **Indy Chef**   ⇆ **Freeway Chef**   ✿ **Country Road Chef**

Oven Baking, Roasting and Moist Braising

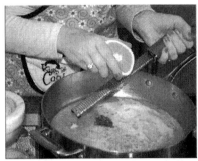

Of all our modern appliances the oven is the unsung hero of the kitchen. With the turn of a dial this single device becomes the vehicle for all manner of cooking, the most important of which are baking, roasting, and moist braising our *Protein First* meals. With minimal preparation and planning we can place a meal in the oven and leave it to be, turning our attention to other matters while the oven does the work. Soon the home is filled with fragrant aromas signaling mealtime is near.

Our high protein diet is easily supported with meals from the oven. Baking, roasting, and braising produce moist protein and lots of it if we chose. A beautifully roasted chicken or turkey will provide many lean protein meals and moist braised meat is always a welcome change.

Braising: The Cooking Vessel

Braising or moist cooking can happen in different vessels including a Dutch oven, the slow cooker, and oven cooking bags. All of these create a tightly closed environment in which simmering liquid vaporizes into steam that swirls around the pot and cooks the meat and vegetables. As the meat and vegetables cook they release flavorful juices that mix with the cooking liquid and soon all of the flavors homogenize in a rich full-flavored meal. All of this happens without interference from the cook, who turns out looking like a culinary rock star when serving a thoughtfully composed well-braised meal.

The braising pot needs to be heavy so that it conducts heat slowly and evenly. Whether braising for long or short durations the pot needs to be heavy, suited to the ingredients holding them snugly, and fitted with a heavy secure lid.

Enamel coated cast-iron Dutch oven is the vessel of preference for many home cooks when it comes to braising. The heavy cooking pot, almost always sized at 7-quarts, is large enough for big cuts of meat such as shoulder roasts, and maintains a tight seal to produce the perfect moist braising environment. Be aware that once filled with ingredients these pots do take some muscle to maneuver: use caution when removing a large heavy pot from the hot oven. The Dutch oven is convenient for recipes that require stove-top cooking of some ingredients as a precursor step before the long oven braising. The Dutch oven easily transfers from stove to oven and back again if the method requires it.

Some cooks use a heavy-gauge 12-inch stainless steel skillet with a tight fitting lid for their braising needs. The skillet should be high sided to come above the ingredients and maintain space for steam and vapor. The stainless steel holds heat very well and can effectively produce a well-braised meal.

Oven Cooking Bags

Oven Bags are a boon to the home cook and I'm surprised we don't reach for them more often, instead reserving them for holiday turkeys and hams. For everyday meals oven roasting protein and vegetables in a cooking bag produces a moist meal in less time than conventional cooking with minimal clean-up. Reynolds® Oven Bags are available in many sizes year round. Originally marketed as "Brown-in-Bag" today's cooking bags are made of transparent, heat-tempered plastic. They are variously sized to cook large turkeys and smaller meals of meat, poultry, pork, often in the company of vegetables and sauce. A cooking bag produces even cooking in less time than using a conventional roasting pan alone.

The method for use is the same for all cooking bag meals: shake flour in the bag, place food in the bag, seal with nylon tie, cut vent holes in top of bag, nestle in roasting pan or baking dish, and place in preheated oven and bake according to recipe directions. When the food inside the oven cooking bag is done, the top of the bag must be slit open carefully to avoid burns from the steam. The food should cool a bit and then served directly from the cooking bag. Large birds and roasts should be moved to a cutting board for carving. Cooking bag meals fit in the moist braised category.

Moist Cooking: Slow Cooker Method

Slow cooker cooking came into favor in the United States when the electric appliance was mass-marketed under the brand name Crock-Pot® manufactured at that time by The Rival Company. The timing was perfect as women were leaving full time homemaking to join the outside-the-home workforce. Meals could be assembled in the slow cooker in the morning and ready for dinner when the family came in the door at the end of the day. The popularity of the slow cooker continues today although most home cooks rely on the device for a few stand-by recipes such as soups and stews without venturing into more creative meals.

For people with weight loss surgery eating a high protein diet and following the liquid restrictions, slow cooker cooking is ideal. Slow cooked protein is moist and tender. Flavors from the seasonings, vegetables, and fruits with which it is cooked enhance our eating experience while adding beneficial nutrients, vitamins, minerals, and fiber. And larger quantities of well-prepared slow cooked food make marvelous leftovers so that we may always have something delicious and appropriate to enjoy while supporting our healthy weight loss surgery diet and weight management goals. If you haven't pulled your slow cooker out for a while, go get it and give some of these recipes a try. Learn the methods and take a chance at creating your own *Protein First* moist meaty slow cooker meal.

Helpful Hints: Slow cookers are manufactured in a variety of sizes measured in quarts. For our purposes I specify using a 4-quart slow cooker: this is the most commonly purchased size in the United States and can accommodate recipes making 4 to 6 servings. All of these recipes were tested in two different slow cookers (both 4-quart) by two different cooks and the results were consistently favorable. The smallest slow cookers sold are 1½-quarts making 1 to 2 servings; the largest are 7 quarts making 6 to 9 servings. Adjust the recipes according to your slow cooker size. (The size should be marked on the bottom of the appliance.)

Safety: Slow cookers are designed to be safe when left unattended. The outer heating base may get hot during cooking, but it should not pose a fire hazard. The heating element in the heating base functions at a low wattage and is safe for use on countertops. Do not operate the slow cooker if the cord is damaged or if the appliance has malfunctioned. Always follow the safeguards and instructions described in the owner's manual.

Foods prepared in a slow cooker should be heated to 165°F, the temperature at which bacteria are killed. Refer to the safe cooking temperatures chart on page 181. Follow the recommended cooking times: avoid opening the lid during cooking. Stirring is not necessary unless adding additional ingredients as directed by the recipe.

Moist Tender Traditional Turkey

Over the years I've tried dozens different turkey recipes and all manner of cooking methods to various results. No matter what I've tried I always come back to the holiday cook's best friend: the oven cooking bag. The reward for using this trusty method is a golden bird with crispy skin and moist succulent meat with plenty of drippings for gravy and sauce. And my goodness clean-up is easy! Don't wait for the holidays. Turkey is outstanding lean protein, delicious any time of the year.

Ingredients:

1 Reynolds® Oven Bag, Turkey Size
1 tablespoon all-purpose flour
2 stalks celery, sliced
1 large onion, sliced
1 (12 to 24-pound) turkey, thawed
canola oil

Directions: Position oven rack at lowest level in oven: preheat oven to 350°F. Shake flour in oven bag; place in roasting pan at least 2-inches deep. Add vegetables to oven bag. Remove neck and giblets from turkey. Rinse turkey under cold running water; pat dry. Season cavity with salt and pepper; rub skin with oil and season with salt and pepper. Place turkey in cooking bag atop vegetables; close with nylon tie. Cut six small slits in bag for vents; tuck remaining bag in roasting pan and make certain the bag will not touch heating element. Refer to timing chart provided with cooking bag to bake the turkey: about 3 hours for a 16 to 20-pound turkey. Allow turkey to rest 10 to 15 minutes before carving. Use juices to make sauce or gravy.

Nutrition: A 4-ounce serving of roasted white meat turkey provides 212 calories, 32 grams protein, 8 grams fat, 0 grams carbohydrate. A 3-ounce serving of roasted dark meat turkey provides 170 calories, 26 grams protein, 7 grams fat, and 0 grams carbohydrate.

Turkey and Eggs Chilled Lunch Plate: Plate leftovers in a ready-to-enjoy meal for the next day. A balanced plate: 3 ounces lean roast turkey; 1 hard cooked egg, peeled and cut in half lengthwise; 1 kiwifruit, peeled and quartered; 6 to 8 fresh berries *(shown on front cover).* Store refrigerated until ready-to-eat. Serve chilled with cranberry sauce.

Sunday-School Cheddar Chicken and Vegetables

↬ Indy Chef, one dish meal, no-tending required while it cooks

Toss the frozen ingredients together before Sunday-School and dinner is ready when you get home. But don't wait for Sunday: give this creamy baking bag recipe a try on any weeknight and enjoy the convenience of pantry and freezer ingredients with the ease of baking bag cooking.

Ingredients:

1 Reynolds® large size oven bag

2 tablespoons flour

1 (10-ounce) can Campbell's Healthy Request® Cheddar Cheese Soup

½ cup chicken broth, low sodium

1 (16-ounce) package frozen baby mixed beans and carrots

6 boneless skinless chicken breast halves, frozen

2 cups prepared white rice, warm

1 bunch fresh parsley for garnish

The frozen vegetables available today meet higher standards than ever before and we can confidently include them in our healthy weight management diet after surgery. It takes mere hours from harvest to processing where vegetables are quick steamed and then flash-frozen. Current USDA standards ensure frozen vegetables provide the best possible nutrition, taste, color, and texture.

Directions: Preheat oven to 350°F. Shake flour in oven bag; place in 13x9x2-inch baking pan. In a large mixing bowl stir together soup, chicken broth, and frozen vegetables; transfer to cooking bag spreading evenly. Nestle each frozen chicken breast half in the sauce and vegetables; close bag with tie; cut six ½-inch slits in top. Place bag in preheated oven and bake for 90 minutes or until chicken is tender. Layer rice on serving platter; top with chicken, sauce, and vegetables. Garnish with fresh sprigs parsley. Serve warm.

Nutrition: Serves 6. Each serving provides 322 calories, 31 grams protein, 5 grams fat, 37 grams carbohydrate, 4 grams dietary fiber.

Try This: Plan one chicken breast half per serving. Take advantage of such an easy cooking method with minimal clean-up and toss in a few extra pieces of chicken for a quality protein meal to enjoy later in the week.

Chili Lime Pork with Sweet Potatoes

⇆Freeway Chef, a riot of flavor,
complete meal in one bag

This is a good example of one recipe addressing many taste sensations: savory, sweet, spicy, and tangy. Using a cooking bag produces moist pork and tender sweet potatoes with a complimentary sauce that rounds-out the meal. Sweet potatoes contain natural sugar that can be overly sweet for WLS patients. Enjoy a scant ¼-cup serving and eat 2 bites of protein to every 1 bite of sweet potato, the 2B/1B eating rhythm.

Ingredients:

1 Reynolds® large size oven bag

1 tablespoons flour

3 tablespoons honey

2 tablespoons chili powder

1 lime, remove zest and reserve

1 (2 to 2 ½-pound) pork top loin roast

2 medium sweet potatoes, peeled and quartered

lime wedges for garnish

> *Is it done?* To measure temperature poke instant-read thermometer through cooking bag and insert into thickest part of meat.

Directions: Preheat oven to 325°F. Shake flour in oven bag; place in 13x9x2-inch baking pan. In a small bowl add the honey, chili powder, and lime zest; juice the lime over the bowl for about 1 tablespoon of juice; whisk all ingredients to blend well. Spread half of chili honey over bottom of pork roast; place roast in cooking bag; spread remaining chili honey over top of roast. Arrange sweet potato quarters around roast in an even layer. Close cooking bag with nylon tie; cut six ½-inch slits in top. Bake in preheated oven for 1 to 1½-hour or until meat thermometer reads 145°F. To serve, slice the roast across the grain; plate sliced pork with 2 sweet potato quarters and drizzled with ¼ cup of chili honey sauce. Garnish with lime wedges.

Nutrition: Serves 8. Each serving provides 255 calories, 26 grams protein, 9 grams fat, 19 grams carbohydrate, 3 grams dietary fiber.

Try This: Get a head start by preparing the recipe through closing the bag with nylon tie. Store in refrigerator with a sticky note to the first person home that evening: *"Cut six small slits in cooking bag, place in cold oven, set temperature to 325°F and cook until done to 145°F internal temperature."* Dinner is served!

French Onion Roast Beef

If you appreciate the flavors of classic French onion soup you will love this recipe. The tender beef takes nicely to the flavors from the beef consume and onion soup that makes a rich gravy for the meat and noodles.

Ingredients:

1 Reynolds® large size oven bag

1 tablespoons flour

1 (2 to 3 pound) beef chuck roast

1 teaspoon garlic powder

3 medium yellow onions, sliced ¼-inch thick, sliced into rings

1 (10.5-ounce) can beef consommé

1 (10.5-ounce) can condensed French onion soup

4 cups wide egg noodles, cooked to package directions

Almost every culture has a version of onion soup, probably because onions are readily available throughout the world. The preparation we are familiar with originates in France and gets the rich flavor from beef broth and caramelized onions. Adding a beef roast to the soup increases the protein count taking advantage of the rich flavors and moist cooking method.

Directions: Preheat oven to 325°F. Shake flour in oven bag; place in 13x9x2-inch baking pan. Season roast with garlic powder, salt, and pepper; place in cooking bag. Arrange onion rings around roast in an even layer. In a small bowl stir beef consommé and French onion soup together; pour over roast and onions in cooking bag. Close cooking bag with nylon tie; cut six ½-inch slits in top. Bake in preheated oven for 1 to 1½-hour or until meat thermometer reads 145°F. To serve, remove roast from bag to cutting board and carve slices against the grain. Pour accumulated juices and onions into a large serving bowl. On a plate arrange 3 to 4-ounces roast beef atop ½-cup egg noodles, ladle ½-cup of sauce and onions over meat and noodles.

Nutrition: Serves 8. Each serving provides 383 calories, 25 grams protein, 19 grams fat, 26 grams carbohydrate, 2 grams dietary fiber.

Oven Braised Swedish Meatballs

The traditional flavors of nutmeg, allspice, and cardamom set these meatballs apart from the typical bland meatballs and gravy one might find at an all-you-can-eat buffet. Gently braised in the oven the meat is moist and tender and the sauce is rich and creamy.

Ingredients:

1½ pounds lean ground beef

½ pound lean ground turkey sausage

1 small onion, finely chopped

2 eggs, beaten

1 cup dry bread crumbs

½ cup evaporated milk

¼ teaspoon ground nutmeg

½ teaspoon ground ginger

½ teaspoon ground allspice

¼ teaspoon ground cardamom

1 cup reduced sodium beef broth

½ cup reduced fat sour cream

3 cups wide egg noodles, cooked

> As an Italian might say,
> *Niente sorpresa, ma tante scoperto.*
> "Nothing surprising but so much to discover."

Directions: In a large bowl gently combine ground beef, turkey sausage and onion. Add eggs, bread crumbs, evaporated milk, nutmeg, ginger, allspice and cardamom. Line a rimmed baking sheet with foil and coat with cooking spray. Preheat oven to 400°F. Shape the meat mixture into 1-inch meatballs and arrange on baking sheet. Bake until lightly browned, about 10 minutes. Remove from oven and lower temperature to 350°F. Transfer meatballs and accumulated juices to oven-safe casserole dish with lid, add beef broth; cover and bake until tender, about 30 minutes. Stir in sour cream, leave uncovered and bake 10 minutes longer. Serve warm over hot noodles.

Nutrition: Serves 6. Each serving provides 537 calories, 36 grams protein, 21 grams fat, 25 grams carbohydrate, 1 gram dietary fiber.

Try This: Make smaller meatballs and serve warmed in a chafing dish as an appetizer or hors d' oeuvre.

Braised Chicken with Mushrooms and Pearl Onions

⇄ Freeway Chef, full flavors, light and dark meat chicken, one-pot meal

This braised meal requires two steps to achieve the full flavor that makes it special. The chicken and vegetables are browned in hot oil to sear in flavors and then liquid is added and the meal is finished in the oven. Only one pot is used in the process simplifying clean-up.

Ingredients:

¼ cup all-purpose flour, seasoned with salt and pepper

6 to 8 meaty chicken pieces, skinless, bone-in (breasts, thighs, legs)

2 tablespoons canola oil

1 shallot, chopped

1 (8-ounce) package button mushrooms, trimmed, wiped clean

1 (10-ounce) bag frozen pearl onions, thawed

1 (14-ounce) can reduced sodium chicken broth

2 tablespoons balsamic vinegar

2 tablespoons fresh thyme, plus sprigs for garnish

Directions: Preheat oven to 350°F. Dredge chicken in seasoned flour, set aside. In a large, heavy Dutch oven heat the canola oil over medium high heat. Add the chicken and cook, turning once, until browned on both sides. Transfer to a platter and tent with foil to keep warm. Add the shallot and cook until softened, about 2 minutes. Add mushrooms and continue cooking until browned, 2 to 4 minutes. Stir in pearl onions and cook 2 to 4 minutes, stirring. Add chicken broth and stir bringing up any browned bits. Return chicken to the pot and bring liquid to a boil. Remove from heat, cover, and place pot in preheated oven, bake for 1 hour until chicken is done and vegetables are tender. Stir in vinegar and chopped thyme, season with salt and pepper. Serve vegetable and pan sauce with one or two pieces of chicken. Garnish with thyme sprigs.

Nutrition: Serves 6. Each serving provides 258 calories, 38 grams protein, 8 grams fat, 7 grams carbohydrate, 1 gram dietary fiber.

Try This: For a rustic version add assorted root vegetables including peeled sliced carrots, sweet potatoes, and parsnips.

Baked Cod with White Beans

We usually think of fish for quick skillet cooking methods. But meaty white fish is delicious when braised in a flavorful and aromatic sauce such as this recipe. More than any other fish recipe I get requests for this one the most. Unlike many fish preparations, this recipe does not need a dipping sauce, the flavorful tomato sauce and cooking juices serve this purpose.

Ingredients:

6 (4-ounce) cod fillets or other firm white fish fillets

1 tablespoon canola oil

1 red bell pepper, seeded, cut into strips

1 yellow onion, sliced into rings

2 cloves garlic, minced

1 (14.5-ounce) can stewed tomatoes

1 (15-ounce) can white beans, rinsed and drained

2 tablespoons white wine vinegar

½ teaspoon dried basil

2 teaspoons capers, drained

fresh parsley for garnish

Directions: Preheat oven to 425°F. Coat a medium sized baking dish or casserole dish with cooking spray. Arrange fish in a single layer; season with salt and pepper. Heat the canola oil in a medium skillet over medium high heat; add bell pepper, onions, and garlic and cook until just tender, about 4 minutes. Arrange over fish. Spoon beans evenly over fish and vegetables. Combine tomatoes with white wine vinegar and dried basil and pour evenly over fish and vegetables. Sprinkle with capers. Bake, uncovered, in preheated oven for 20 minutes or until fish is done and flakes easily when tested with fork. Serve warm, 1 filet with 2/3-cup vegetables, beans and sauce. Garnish with fresh parsley.

Nutrition: Serves 6. Each serving provides 228 calories, 27 grams protein, 3 grams fat, 23 grams carbohydrate, 5 grams dietary fiber.

Try This: Use flavored canned tomato blends in place of the stewed tomatoes.

Rustic Oven-Baked Cassoulet

⇆ Freeway Chef, hearty comforting carb-taming meal, one pot method

Cassoulet is a French cooking term for a rich slow-cooked casserole. Typically cassoulet contains poultry, pork, or lamb; sausage for flavor and always white beans. The name comes from the traditional cooking vessel, the *cassole*: a deep round earthenware pot with a lid. While the cassoulet takes effort to compose, once in the oven it is best left unattended, giving the cook a welcome respite from toil over a hot stove.

Ingredients:

1 tablespoon canola oil

6 chicken thighs, bone-in, skinless

1 (8-ounce) package kielbasa, reduced fat, cut in ½-inch slices

½ cup dry white wine

2 medium carrots, thinly sliced

1 medium white onion, cut into thin wedges

1 stalk celery, sliced

2 cloves garlic, minced

1 (14.5-ounce) can diced tomatoes

½ teaspoon Italian seasoning

2 (15-ounce) cans great northern beans, rinsed and drained

Directions: Preheat oven to 350°F. In a large Dutch oven heat canola oil over medium high heat. Add chicken thighs, meaty side down, and brown on both sides, about 10 minutes. Remove to plate, season with salt and pepper, keep warm. Add kielbasa, cook and stir browning slightly. Remove kielbasa to plate with chicken; deglaze Dutch oven with white wine. Add carrots, onion, celery, and garlic, cooking and stirring until vegetables just become tender, about 4 minutes. Add diced tomatoes, Italian Seasoning, and beans; stir well. Arrange chicken thighs, meaty side up, and kielbasa in pot; cover; place in preheated oven. Bake 50 minutes undisturbed until meat chicken is done and liquid is thickened. Taste and adjust seasoning with salt and pepper; serve warm: 1 piece chicken and 1 cup cassoulet per person.

Nutrition: Serves 6. Each serving provides 405 calories, 24 grams protein, 16 grams fat, 38 grams carbohydrate, 9 grams dietary fiber.

Provence-Style Baked Beef and Vegetables

↰ Freeway Chef, unfussy, moist
succulent meat and vegetables

This fantastic braised beef stew deserves the Freeway Chef grade in Pace of Preparation because all ingredients are assembled in one pot, covered, and braised in the oven. This method produces a deeply flavored dish without the extra steps of browning the meat or vegetables.

Ingredients:

¼ cup soy sauce, reduced sodium

1 teaspoon Worcestershire sauce

¼ cup all-purpose flour

2 pounds beef stew meat, cubed

4 carrots, sliced

1 medium yellow onion, sliced

2 ribs celery, sliced

2 cloves garlic, minced

1 teaspoon dried Herbes de Provence seasoning blend

1 cup dry red wine

1 cup beef broth

1 (8-ounce) package button mushrooms

Herbes de Provence is an herbal seasoning typically containing savory, fennel, basil, thyme, and lavender. The blend is favored by chefs composing vegetable stews where the slow cooking infuses the flavor into the cooked food. Before the mixture was commercially blended in the 1970s cooks passed their secret formula from one family generation to the next. Some families deeply guarded their herbal blend secret formula, much to the angst of rival families and cooks.

Directions: Preheat oven to 325°F. In a large Dutch oven whisk together soy sauce, Worcestershire sauce, and flour. Add beef and toss to coat; season with salt and pepper. Stir in remaining ingredients: carrots, onion, celery, garlic, herb blend, red wine, beef broth, and mushrooms. Cover and place Dutch oven in preheated oven. Bake undisturbed for 90 minutes. Remove from oven, stir well and ladle 1½-cup serving per person. Serve with Mashed Garlic Cauliflower, page 127.

Nutrition: Serves 8. Each serving provides 268 calories, 32 grams protein, 8 grams fat, 10 grams carbohydrate, 2 grams dietary fiber.

Try This: Prepare stew and place in oven before an evening outing and come home to a perfectly braised meal ready to serve.

Old Dutch Pork with Cabbage

The Pennsylvania Dutch settlers took great pride in their farm raised pork, apple orchards, and garden produce. This traditional pork and cabbage stew was typical food served at harvest celebrations in early colonial times. More adventurous cooks may wish to use hard apple cider in place of the apple cider for greater depth of flavor.

Ingredients:

1½ pounds pork shoulder

1 tablespoon canola oil

1 tablespoon butter

2 medium yellow onions, chopped

1 medium granny Smith apple, peeled, chopped

1 (1-pound) green cabbage shredded

½ teaspoon caraway seeds

1 cup apple cider

Directions: Preheat oven to 325°F. Trim pork and cut into bite size pieces; season with salt and pepper. In a large Dutch oven heat the canola oil and butter over medium high heat; add the pork and cook and stir until browned on all sides. Add the onion; cook and stir 4 minutes until onion starts to become tender and aromatic. Stir in apple, cabbage, caraway seed, and apple cider. Cover Dutch oven, place in preheated oven. Bake undisturbed for 90 minutes. Test pork for doneness, it should be fork tender; and adjust seasoning with salt and pepper. Ladle into soup mugs or bowls and serve warm with rustic bread.

Nutrition: Serves 8. Each serving provides 270 calories, 19 grams protein, 16 grams fat, 12 grams carbohydrate, 2 grams dietary fiber.

Try This: For added seasoning and flavor include 8 ounces of pork sausage in this stew, cutting into ½-inch pieces and browning with pork meat. ~ Prepare wide egg noodles following package directions, drain, sauté in butter with ½ teaspoon caraway seeds, ladle pork stew over noodles.

Holiday Prime Rib Roast of Beef

☼ **Country Road Chef**

We have a tradition of cooking and serving a prime rib roast of beef for Christmas Eve Dinner. The occasion calls for grand extravagance and the prime rib roast with its grand cost and grand presence fits the menu perfectly. Because I only cook such a roast once a year it is critical to have a fail-proof recipe; there is simply no room for error. With a few minor adjustments I follow the method in Barbara Kafka's *Roasting: A Simple Art* and it produces consistently good results worthy of the most extravagant table we set all year.

Ingredients:

1 (6 to 10 pound) standing rib roast
1 clove garlic per pound of roast
kosher salt and black pepper
1 (14.5-ounce) can beef broth
1 (750ml) bottle dry red wine
1 (8-ounce) container sour cream
1 tablespoon creamy horseradish
1 bunch parsley for garnish

SNAP!

Pictured on Front Cover

Directions: Unwrap roast and position on rack in roaster pan; allow to sit at room temperature one hour, covered with a loosely woven clean kitchen towel. Slice garlic thinly and tuck in roast under fat layer, distributing it evenly. Season roast generously with kosher salt and black pepper; pour beef broth and one-half the red wine in bottom of roaster. Position oven rack on lowest level; preheat oven to 500°F. Place roast in oven and cook 45 minutes (oven may give off some smoke from cooking). Without opening oven lower temperature to 325°F and continue cooking 5 minutes per pound (about 30 to 50 minutes). Raise oven temperature to 500°F and cook 15 minutes longer. Internal temperature should be 135°F on an instant-read thermometer: return to oven if necessary to reach this temperature. Move roast to carving board, tent with foil, allow to rest 10 to 15 minutes. Deglaze roasting pan with remaining red wine, strain liquid through fine mesh sieve and serve au jus with roast. While roast cooks mix sour cream and horseradish into smooth sauce to serve with meat.   Carve roast into 1-inch thick slices and serve with au jus and horseradish cream, garnished with parsley.

Nutrition: Serves many. Each 4-ounce serving provides 454 calories, 26 grams protein, 38 grams fat, 0 grams carbohydrate, 0 grams dietary fiber.

Gentleman Joes on English Muffins

⇆Freeway Chef, family friendly,
perfect for buffet or tailgating

In a play on words I call these open faced sandwiches Gentleman Joes to avoid confusion with a distant culinary cousin called Sloppy Joe. The meaty sauce in our more genteel version is served on toasted English muffin halves and civilly enjoyed with a fork and knife. It's not just good manners in play here, however. Studies suggest that meals eaten slowly with utensils versus quickly out of hand, create a better sensory experience and feelings of satisfaction are prolonged.

Ingredients:
½ cup ketchup
½ cup barbecue sauce
2 tablespoons apple cider vinegar
1 tablespoon brown sugar
1 teaspoon chili powder
1 tablespoon Worcestershire sauce
1 (14.5-ounce) can baked beans
1 tablespoon canola oil
1½ pounds 95% lean ground beef
1 small onion, chopped
1 red bell pepper, chopped
1 clove garlic, minced
3 English Muffins, split and toasted
6 (1-ounce) slices Cheddar cheese

Browning meat before adding it to a slow cooker adds color and flavor. But if you're in a hurry, you can skip this step – *EXCEPT* for ground meat. Browning ground meat helps remove fat, keeps the pieces from clumping, and sears the meat with appetizing color. It allows unattended slow cooking because there is no need for stirring to break-up the ground meat as it cooks.

Directions: Combine the ketchup, barbecue sauce, apple cider vinegar, brown sugar, Worcestershire sauce, and baked beans in a 4-quart slow cooker. Heat canola oil in a large skillet over medium high heat; add ground beef, onion, bell pepper, and garlic and cook stirring to break up meat; season beef with salt and pepper. Drain and discard excess fat. Add meat mixture to slow cooker and stir with sauce and beans to combine. Cover; set cooker to high and cook 3 hours; or set cooker to low and cook 5 hours. Serve ½ cup Gentleman Joe meat mixture on ½ toasted English muffin topped with one slice of Cheddar.

Nutrition: Serves 6. Each serving provides 583 calories, 25 grams protein, 13 grams fat, 40 grams carbohydrate, 7 grams dietary fiber.

Beef Puttanesca over Noodles

Traditional puttanesca sauce is a spicy blend of tomatoes, onions, anchovies, oregano, and garlic cooked with olive oil. The Italian sauce is generally served with pasta and garlic is the dominant flavor and fragrance.

Ingredients:

1 tablespoon olive oil

1 pound 95% lean ground beef

1 large yellow onion, chopped

4 cloves garlic, minced

1 teaspoon anchovy paste

1 teaspoon Italian seasoning blend

¼ teaspoon crushed red pepper flakes

2 (14.5-ounce) cans diced tomatoes

1 (6-ounce) can tomato paste

1 (8-ounce) package multigrain pasta

1 bunch fresh parsley, for garnish

> Anchovy Paste is an appealing combination of pounded anchovies, vinegar, spices and water. A small amount adds salty-savory flavor without overpowering a dish. Find anchovy paste by the canned anchovies in your grocery store or look for it in gourmet specialty shops.

Directions: Heat olive oil in a large skillet over medium high heat. Add ground beef, cook and stir breaking apart meat as it browns. Add onion, minced garlic, anchovy paste, Italian seasoning, and red pepper flakes to meat; stir to combine. Place meat in a 4-quart slow cooker, stir-in tomatoes and tomato paste. Cover; set cooker to high and cook 4 hours; or set cooker to low and cook 6 hours. About 20 minutes before serving prepare pasta according to package directions. Serve ½ cup sauce over ½ cup of pasta. Garnish with parsley.

Nutrition: Serves 8. Each serving provides 262 calories, 19 grams protein, 8 grams fat, 30 grams carbohydrate, 5 grams dietary fiber.

Try This: In place of the ground beef use frozen Italian seasoned meatballs from the freezer section at your market. Simply add frozen meatballs to slow cooker, omitting the browning step, and follow the recipe as directed. Using meatballs speeds the assembly process while making the meal feel extra special.

The slow cooker is a cozy home for the traditional layers of lasagna and makes a convenient vessel for serving this hot meal at a potluck gathering.

Ingredients:

1 (12-ounce) Krinkly Egg Noodles from American Beauty®

10 ounces Jennie-O® Lean Sweet Italian Turkey Sausage

1¼ pounds extra lean ground beef

1 yellow onion, diced

2 cloves garlic, minced

1 tablespoon tomato paste

1 tablespoon red wine vinegar

2 cups prepared spaghetti sauce

1 (15-ounce) container ricotta cheese

½ cup grated Parmesan cheese

2 tablespoons fresh Italian parsley, minced

2 cups mozzarella cheese, grated, divided

When hosting a gathering where many warm food dishes are served consider the slow cooker your go-to appliance for casseroles, sauces, or stews. This makes space on the stove or in the oven for other dishes.

Directions: Lightly spritz the stoneware bowl of the slow cooker with olive oil flavored cooking spray; set aside. Cook Krinkly Egg Noodles for half the time directed on package; drain; set aside. While noodles cook, in a large skillet over high heat, brown ground beef and turkey sausage mixing together as they cook. Add onion and garlic; continue cooking 2 to 3 minutes until fragrant. Remove from heat, add tomato paste, red wine vinegar, and spaghetti sauce; stir well to combine. In a medium bowl fold together the ricotta, Parmesean, and minced parsley; set aside. Place 1/3 of beef mixture in bottom of slow cooker; top with half of the partially cooked krinkly noodles, half ricotta mixture and ½ cup mozzarella cheese. Repeat layers ending with a third layer of meat. Cover; cook on low without stirring for 3 to 4 hours or high without stirring for 2 to 3 hours. About 30 minutes before serving remove cover, distribute remaining 1 cup mozzarella over lasagna. Return cover, turn off heat, and let casserole sit 20 to 30 minutes to make serving easier

Nutrition: Serves 8 to 10. Each serving provides approximately 514 calories, 31 grams protein, 35 grams fat, 26 grams carbohydrate, 3 grams dietary fiber.

Slow Cooker Tri-Color Pepper Steak

⇆ **Freeway Chef, American Classic,
colorful peppers provide antioxidants**

My grandmother Flo frequently served pepper steak using only green peppers and grandpa complained that he disliked the dish. The funny thing, he always cleaned his plate and usually had a second serving. I prefer red, yellow, or orange peppers for their milder flavor and pretty presentation.

Ingredients:

2 tablespoons canola oil

3 pounds beef round steak, cut into strips

4 cloves garlic, minced

1 large onion, chopped

½ cup soy sauce, reduced sodium

2 teaspoons brown sugar

½ teaspoon ground ginger

1 each red, yellow, and green bell pepper, cut into strips

1 package instant wild rice

¼ cup cold water

1 tablespoon cornstarch

Use the color of peppers you prefer and enjoy this easy dish often: it provides many health-promoting nutrients. Red bell peppers are simply ripened green pepper and supply 11 times the beta carotene of a green pepper. A red bell pepper contains four times as much vitamin C as an orange.

Directions: Heat canola oil in a large skillet over medium high heat. Add half steak strips, cook and stir until browned; place in 4-quart slow cooker. Cook remaining half of steak strips, stir in garlic, onion, soy sauce, brown sugar, and ground ginger. Add to slow cooker and stir well. Cover and cook on low for 6 to 8 hours or high 4 to 6 hours or until meat is tender. One hour before serving add bell pepper strips, stirring well. Prepare instant rice following package directions. In a small bowl whisk together water and cornstarch; add to steak mixture and cook uncovered, on high for 15 minutes for sauce to thicken. Serve pepper steak atop rice.

Nutrition: Serves 8: ½-cup rice; 1 cup Pepper Steak. Per serving: 374 calories, 42 grams protein, 15 grams fat, 17 grams carbohydrate, 2 grams dietary fiber.

Try This: Pepper Steak also prepares well in a skillet if you don't have time for the slow cooker. Brown meat with garlic and onions; cover and simmer until tender before adding pepper slices and thickening sauce.

Autumn's Best Beef and Beer Casserole

⇄ Freeway Chef, affordable comfort
food, cooked all-day richness

Beef stew meat is a less expensive cut and can be tough; the beer in this recipe serves to tenderize the meat. Chose a medium stout beer for the best flavor: light beer will contribute little flavor and dark beer may be too heavy or bitter.

Ingredients:

2 tablespoons canola oil

2 pounds cubed beef stew meat

1½-teaspoon all-purpose seasoning

2 tablespoons all-purpose flour

1 cup beef broth

1 (12-ounce) bottle brown ale or beer

1 cup water

1 white onion, sliced

2 carrots, sliced

2 stalks celery, sliced

2 to 3 cloves garlic, peeled, crushed

1 (8-ounce) package button mushrooms, sliced

1 sweet potato, peeled, cut into 1-inch cubes

Even in the busiest lives there are days when we

must
        slow
                down.

Slow cooker meals let the time we save in the kitchen become ours to savor at the table enjoying a healthy meal with people we love. Let's take our time.
        Let's slow down.

Directions: Heat canola oil in a large skillet over medium high heat. Add stew meat and cook and stir browning on all sides. Season with all-purpose seasoning; and salt and pepper: spoon beef into slow cooker; leaving oil and drippings in skillet. Return skillet to heat; add flour and whisk to blend; cook 1 minute. Slowly add beef broth and beer to skillet, whisking to combine and blend into a smooth sauce. Bring to a boil and cook for 2 minutes to thicken and reduce; add to slow cooker. Add onion, carrots, celery, garlic, mushrooms, and sweet potato. Stir well, cover, set cooker to high and cook 4 to 6 hours or set to low and cook 8 to 10 hours. Stir well before serving. Casserole should be moist and thick.

Nutrition: Serves 6 to 8. Each 1½-cup serving provides 398 calories, 42 grams protein, 16 grams fat, 17 grams carbohydrate, 3 grams dietary fiber.

Note:

Ingredients:

Directions:

Nutrition:

Slow Cooked Creamy Chicken and Mushrooms

↹Freeway Chef, extreme comfort
food, delicious easy leftovers

This is an unbeatable combination of flavors, texture, and nutrients. Who wouldn't be happy after a long day of work and the rat-race to come home and enjoy this meal knowing it tastes good and provides healthy nutrients?

Ingredients:

1 teaspoon all-purpose seasoning blend

½ teaspoon paprika

2 pounds boneless skinless chicken breasts and/or thighs

1 (8-ounce) package button mushrooms, sliced

1 medium sweet onion, sliced

1 (14.5-ounce) can chicken broth, reduced sodium

1 tablespoon cornstarch

1 cup sour cream

2 cups hot cooked rice

fresh parsley sprigs for garnish

> Sweet onions include Vidalia, Maui, Walla Walla, and Granex. At the market look for dry (long storage) onions with crisp, papery skins. Store in a cool dark space in an open container; do not store in sealed plastic bags or containers. Discard any onion that begins to sprout.

Directions: Thaw chicken pieces if frozen. Season chicken with all-purpose seasoning blend, paprika, and salt and pepper: place in 4-quart slow cooker. Top with sliced mushrooms and onions; add chicken broth. Cover and set slow cooker on high for 3 hours or low for 5 to 6 hours. Prepare rice following package directions. Transfer chicken and vegetables to platter; cover with foil to keep warm. Carefully pour 2 cups cooking liquid into small saucepan set over high heat and whisk in the cornstarch. Continue whisking and bring to a boil, cooking and whisking until liquid thickens to gravy consistency. Remove from heat and let cool about 5 minutes. Whisk in sour cream. Serve chicken over rice drenched in creamy sauce and garnished with parsley.

Nutrition: Serves 6. Each serving provides 378 calories, 40 grams protein, 12 grams fat, 25 grams carbohydrate, 1 gram dietary fiber.

Rustic Chicken Cacciatore

Cacciatore is a traditional hunter's stew made of poultry with vegetables including onions and mushrooms simmered in tomato sauce. Using prepared marinara sauce makes this recipe simple and delicious. Rather than serve this meal with rustic bread or pasta try serving it with spaghetti squash for a healthy low-carb alternative that suits our *Protein First* diet.

Ingredients:

1 (26 to 32-ounce) jar prepared commercial or homemade marinara sauce

1 (6-ounce) can tomato paste

¼ cup dry red wine or chicken broth

1 teaspoon Italian herb seasoning blend

2 pounds chicken thighs, bone-in, skinless

1 small yellow onion, sliced

2 cloves garlic, peeled, smashed

1 (8-ounce) package button mushrooms, cleaned and quartered

1 (3 to 4 pound) spaghetti squash

½ cup grated Parmesan cheese

> Once a slow cooker meal is in progress avoid lifting the lid as much as possible to prevent heat loss. Unless the recipe directions state otherwise, stirring during slow cooking is unnecessary.

Directions: With a wooden spoon stir together marinara sauce, tomato paste, wine or chicken broth, and seasoning blend in a 4-quart slow cooker. Nestle chicken thighs in sauce; top with sliced onions, smashed garlic cloves, and button mushrooms. Cover and cook on high 3 to 4 hours or set to low and cook 6 to 8 hours. About 40 minutes before serving prepare spaghetti squash as directed on page 138. Serve 1 chicken thigh with ½ cup vegetables and sauce on top of ½ cup spaghetti squash sprinkled with 1 to 2 tablespoons Parmesan cheese.

Nutrition: Serves 6-8. Each serving provides 259 calories, 26 grams protein, 9 grams fat, 22 grams carbohydrate, 4 grams dietary fiber.

Try This: Serve over baked mashed butternut squash for an equally delicious meal full of beta carotene, vitamins A and C, and dietary fiber.

Pasta and Rice: Measured Portions Matter

Many weight loss surgery patients report they are told to exclude pasta, rice, polenta, couscous, etc. (simple starch) from their diet following weight loss surgery. The reasoning is that these simple starches take up too much pouch volume without providing sufficient nutritional value to justify the space-investment. And let's be honest: it is likely we ate too much of these low-nutrient starchy foods before surgery which contributed to our morbid obesity. Complete exclusion of specific foods seldom works very long with any dietary management effort. Over the years I have learned that including pasta or rice as a controlled and measured ingredient in a meal actually works with our weight management program and may prevent unchecked eating of other non-nutritional starchy carbohydrates. That is why I include pasta and rice in small measured quantities as part of my WLS diet, as you see in some recipes within this book.

Small Measured Quantities: This is key. I know it is annoying to measure rice or pasta portions. It is for me and I've heard from enough people in our WLS Neighborhood to know we *all* find it a hassle. The best way I can state this is that if we cannot be bothered to measure our pasta serving tonight, then tomorrow morning when we step on the bathroom scale we should not be bothered when the results are not what we hoped for. Measuring food portions is as important in our weight management as measuring body weight. They are intrinsically related. We tend to be polarized by one measurement (body weight) and ambivalent to the other measurement (food portions) when in fact one directly affects the other.

Weight loss surgery patients are pro-active people by nature. We took pro-active measures to alter the course of our illness, morbid obesity, by having gastric surgery. We can achieve the best results – *the results that motivated us to pursue a surgical option* – when we routinely measure and monitor our food intake. A hyper-awareness of what and how much we eat will certainly give us the results we desire on that other revered symbol of measurement: the bathroom scale.

As always, follow the dietary program prescribed by your bariatric center; your general care physician; and/or your nutritionist. Seek their advice when making significant dietary changes.

Pasta & Rice – Simple Starches Measured Portions Matter				
¼-Cup Serving-Cooked Ready-to-Eat	Calories	Protein (grams)	Carbohydrates (grams)	Fiber (grams)
Spaghetti	49	2	10	1
Whole wheat pasta	44	2	10	1
Egg noodles	53	2	10	Trace
Angel Hair	46	2	8	1
Couscous	44	1	9	1
Soba noodles	48	2	11	0
White rice	60	1	13	Trace
Brown rice	55	1	9	1
Wild rice	41	2	9	1
Polenta	41	1	9	1

As you can see, a ¼-cup serving of pasta or rice is does not contain a worrisome amount of calories or carbohydrates. After much experimentation I know that ¼-cup is my perfect serving. It gives me enough pasta taste and texture to satisfy cravings without taking up too much pouch space or causing weight gain. If you don't know your perfect pasta serving I suggest you start with a ¼-cup serving and make the following observation:

- Does this serving satisfy my desire for pasta with this meal?
- Is my meal *Protein First*? (See page 21: Protein First)
- Do I find myself wanting more pasta?
- Do I notice weight gain after eating this portion of pasta with a *Protein First* meal?

Once you conduct deliberate and calculated experimentation you will be able to successfully include simple starch in your diet in a nutritionally positive manner. The small action of measuring portions and learning what works for your body will be rewarded when you monitor the other measurement in which we invest so much meaning: body weight. Use the table on the following page to discover your perfect pasta portion:

Pasta & Rice – Simple Starches
My Perfect Portion

Date: Meal (B, L, D*)	Type of Starch	Serving Size	Satisfying? Yes/No	Protein First? Yes/No	Want More? Yes/No
Notes:					
Notes:					
Notes:					
Notes:					
Notes:					
Notes:					

*Breakfast, Lunch, Dinner

Use the data you've collected above to determine your perfect pasta portion. Be open to change over the progression of your weight loss surgery post-op lifetime. Continue to collect information and make adjustments so that your diet is working with you in meeting your weight management goals. Download this and many other free forms at LivingAfterWLS.com – Click Downloads.

Shredded Salsa Chicken

If you always keep a bag of frozen chicken breasts and a jar of salsa on hand you have the makings of an emergency meal. This is a workday standby for me and nobody ever complains when I serve shredded salsa chicken wrapped in a tortilla. Put out a bagged green salad and some taco toppings and serve up a fiesta!

Ingredients:

6 to 8 chicken breast halves, boneless, skinless, frozen

1 (16-ounce) jar prepared salsa

> Using frozen boneless skinless chicken is not only convenient, it gives good results. Following directed cooking times the chicken is tender without being mushy and overcooked.

Directions: Make certain chicken breasts are still frozen, but not stuck together. Pour about half of the prepared salsa in the bottom of slow cooker. Layer chicken breasts on salsa. Pour remaining salsa on chicken breasts. Cover slow cooker and set to low; cook 6 to 8 hours or set to high; cook 3 to 4 hours until chicken is tender and can be pulled apart with forks. Remove chicken breasts to a rimmed pan or plate and pull chicken with forks to make shredded chicken. Place in serving bowl. With a slotted spoon scoop solids from slow cooker adding to chicken. Mix adding enough cooking liquid to reach desired moisture and consistency. Use shredded salsa chicken as a filling for tacos, enchiladas, wraps, chicken salad, a simple protein with rice, or topping for a tossed salad. Once cooked and cooled the shredded salsa chicken may be packaged for individual servings and frozen for future meals.

Nutrition: Each 4-ounce serving provides 190 calories, 35 grams protein, 1 gram fat, 5 grams carbohydrate, trace dietary fiber.

Try This: For added fiber and vegetable protein add one (15-ounce) can black beans, rinsed and drained, to shredded chicken. ~ Use Shredded Salsa Chicken to build a taco pizza: layer chicken with refried beans, cheese, olives, green onions, tomatoes on a ready-to-eat pizza crust. Bake as directed; serve warm with guacamole, sour cream, and salsa.

Turkey Tenderloin Paprikash with Egg Noodles

With the increasing availability of fresh turkey and turkey parts, such as the tenderloin in this recipe, we have more opportunities to include this healthy protein in our menu rotation.

Ingredients:

1 (20-ounce) turkey tenderloin

2 tablespoons all-purpose flour

¼ teaspoon salt

¼ teaspoon pepper

1 teaspoon Hungarian paprika

¼ teaspoon red pepper flakes

2 tablespoons canola oil

1 small onion, chopped

1 clove garlic, minced

1 (14.5-ounce) can diced tomatoes

1 (12-ounce) package egg noodles

¼ cup sour cream

1 bunch parsley, for garnish

Paprika is a powder made by grinding aromatic sweet red pepper pods: the flavor varies from mild and sweet to pungent and hot. Freshly ground paprika can be bright orange-red to deep blood-red. Most commercial paprika comes from Spain, South America, California, and Hungary. Many chefs consider Hungarian paprika superior to all others and will include "Hungarian" in the name of any dish that features this seasoning.

Directions: Slice turkey tenderloin into 8 equal pieces. If necessary pound with meat mallet so all are approximately the same thickness. With a fork stir together flour, salt, pepper, paprika, and pepper flakes on a pie plate. Dredge each turkey tenderloin cutlet in flour to coat both sides. In a large skillet heat oil over medium high heat until hot. Add turkey in a single layer and brown both sides of each cutlet. Place cutlets in 4-quart slow cooker. Add onion and garlic to skillet, cook and stir until onion begins to soften and turn golden. Add to slow cooker; stir in tomatoes. Cover; cook on low 1 to 2 hours. Twenty minutes before serving prepare noodles following package directions. Serve warm noodles topped with two turkey cutlets and 1/3 cup onion and tomato sauce. Top with sour cream and garnish with parsley.

Nutrition: Serves 4. Each serving provides 352 calories, 35 grams protein, 12 grams fat, 25 grams carbohydrate, 2 grams dietary fiber.

**☞Indy Chef, tender beefy morsels,
creamy paprika sauce, easy preparation**

This recipe does not require the beef to be browned before placing in the slow cooker. However, if you have time and enjoy the added flavor then brown the beef in 2 tablespoons of hot canola oil after it has been dusted with the seasoned flour.

Ingredients:

2 pounds beef round steak

2 tablespoons all-purpose flour

1½-teaspoon Hungarian paprika

¼ teaspoon dried thyme

1 bay leaf

1 large onion, coarsely chopped

1 clove garlic, peeled and minced

1 (14.5-ounce) can diced tomatoes

1 (12-ounce) package wide egg noodles

1 cup sour cream

For some in this country the word goulash has come to mean a *mish'mash* of leftovers best left unnamed. The word goulash, however, is actually Hungarian for a stew made of beef or other meat and vegetables and flavored with Hungarian paprika.

Directions: Trim steak of fat and cut into 1-inch cubes; season with salt and pepper; set aside. In a 1-gallon zip-top plastic bag place flour, Hungarian paprika, and dried thyme. Working in small batches shake beef cubes in seasoned flour; place in slow cooker and continue until all beef is dusted with flour. Top meat with bay leaf, diced onion and minced garlic; add tomatoes; stir once to combine ingredients. Cover and set slow cooker to low; cook for 8 to 10 hours or set to high and cook 4 to 5 hours until beef is tender. About 30 minutes before serving prepare egg noodles following package directions. Just before serving remove bay leaf; add sour cream to beef and stir well to blend. Serve beef over warm egg noodles.

Nutrition: Serves 6 (2/3-cup beef with 1/3 cup egg noodles). Each serving provides 318 calories, 29 grams protein, 14 grams fat, 15 grams carbohydrate, 1 gram dietary fiber.

Try This: For a tailgate or potluck stir warm noodles into beef and sauce; set cooker to low and serve directly from slow cooker buffet style. Serve with additional sour cream on the side and paprika for garnish.

Turkey Filled Colorful Peppers

⇆Freeway Chef, delectable aroma, low carbs, high nutrients, low calories

Oven-baked stuffed peppers require the ground meat be cooked in a skillet before the peppers are stuffed and baked. Slow cooker stuffed peppers eliminate this step while producing a moist meaty *Protein First* meal.

Ingredients:

3 sweet bell peppers; assorted colors

1 (20-ounce) package Jennie-O® Lean Ground Turkey Breast

1 small onion, minced

1 carrot, grated

1 stalk celery, minced

1½ teaspoons Mrs. Dash® Original Seasoning

¼ teaspoon ground pepper

1 egg

1 (8-ounce) can tomato sauce

1 to 2 cups chicken broth, reduced sodium

3 ounces shredded Monterey Jack

We often associate slow cooker meals with fall and winter. But consider using the slow cooker year-round. In the spring and summer fresh vegetables are abundant and the cooker does the work without heating-up the kitchen like using the oven or stove does.

Directions: Wash and dry bell peppers. Depending upon how peppers will fit in your slow cooker remove stems and cut vertically so each pepper half will rest on its side; or cut top off so peppers will rest upright. Remove seeds and membranes; set aside. In a medium mixing bowl gently mix the ground turkey, onion, carrot, celery, seasoning blend, ground pepper, egg, and tomato sauce. Spoon mixture evenly in peppers; arrange peppers in slow cooker; add enough chicken broth to fill bottom of cooker 1 to 2-inches deep. Cover; set cooker to low and cook 4 to 6 hours or high and cook 2 to 4 hours. About 30 minutes before serving check meat for doneness using an instant-read meat thermometer: temperature should be 160°F. If turkey is done top peppers with cheese; return cover and continue cooking 10 to 15 minutes until cheese is melted. Serve warm.

Nutrition: Serves 6. Each serving provides 201 calories, 29 grams protein, 6 grams fat, 6 grams carbohydrate, 1 gram dietary fiber.

Try This: Prepare 2 cups cooked white rice and serve with stuffed peppers.

Smothered Pork Chops

⇆ **Freeway Chef, moist meaty flavors,
weeknight family meal**

Smothered pork chops are moist and succulent taking on the flavors of the ingredients with which they are prepared. This moist preparation works well for a WLS high-protein diet because the balance of protein to complex carbohydrates is achieved with interesting flavors and palatable textures.

Ingredients:

4 slices thick-cut bacon

6 bone-in pork chops, trimmed of fat

1 teaspoon all-purpose seasoning blend

1 tablespoon butter

2 onions, sliced ¼-inch thick rings

2 cloves garlic, minced

1 tablespoons brown sugar

¼ cup soy sauce, reduced sodium

1 cup chicken broth, reduced sodium

1 tablespoon apple cider vinegar

1½ cups warm cooked white rice

fresh parsley sprigs for garnish

> For Apricot Smothered Pork Chops add ¾-cup chopped dried apricots to onion mixture with 1 (11-ounce) jar apricot preserves in place of the soy sauce and broth. Follow recipe as otherwise directed and enjoy! Apricots are a good source of potassium and a flavorful compliment to pork.

Directions: In a large skillet cook bacon over medium high heat until crisp; drain on paper towels; crumble into bottom of 4-quart slow cooker. Season pork chops with salt and pepper and all-purpose seasoning blend; working in batches brown chops in bacon drippings; add to slow cooker layering as necessary. Melt butter in skillet; add onions, garlic, and brown sugar; cook and stir until onions release juices and start to become tender. Transfer onions to slow cooker leaving drippings and bits in skillet. Deglaze skillet by whisking soy sauce, broth, and vinegar together over high heat; when reduced add juice to slow cooker. Cover; set to low and cook 5 to 6 hours or set to high and cook 3 to 4 hours. Serve 1 pork chop with ¼-cup rice smothered with ¼ to ½-cup onions. Garnish with fresh parsley sprigs.

Nutrition: Serves 6. Each serving provides 403 calories, 23 grams protein, 25grams fat, 21 grams carbohydrate, 1 gram dietary fiber

Autumnal Pork Roast Slow-Cooked Meal

✿Country Road Chef, slow cooked flavors, big beautiful autumnal meal

Pork shoulder roast contains more fat than pork tenderloin making it a perfect cut for slow cooker braising. This is an ideal Sunday dinner in fall and winter when root vegetables, apples, and cranberries are abundant. I call this a ✿Country Road Chef meal because taking time to prepare the vegetables and later enjoy the meal is part of the pleasure.

Ingredients:

2 large white onions, peeled and quartered

3 stalks celery, cut into 2-inch pieces

1 sweet potato, peeled, cut into 8 wedges

1 green apple, cored, cut into 8 wedges

¼ cup light brown sugar

1½ teaspoon poultry seasoning*

1 teaspoon salt

½ teaspoon pepper

3 pounds pork butt roast, trimmed, cut into 2 to 3-inch chunks

1 cup fresh whole cranberries

2 tablespoons butter, cut into 8 pieces

1 cup chicken broth

Apple slices and fresh cranberries for garnish

> In slow cooking do not increase liquid over the measurement specified in the recipe. Slow cooking releases and retains more juices from meats and vegetables than in conventional cooking.

Directions: Layer onions, celery, sweet potato, and apple wedges in a 4-quart slow cooker. In a large mixing bowl blend the brown sugar, poultry seasoning, salt, and pepper. Add the pork chunks; toss to coat. Place seasoned pork on vegetables in slow cooker; top with cranberries, and dot with butter pieces. Add chicken broth; cover slow cooker; set to low and cook 8 to 10 hours or high and cook 6 to 8 hours. Arrange pork, vegetables and fruit on serving platter. Drizzle with juices; garnish with fresh apple slices and cranberries. Serve warm to the happy people lucky to be at your table for such a grand meal.

*Look for poultry blend made of ground sage, thyme, savory, and celery salt.

Nutrition: Serves 6 to 8. Each serving provides approximately 512 calories, 36 grams protein, 30 grams fat, 25 grams carbohydrate, 3 grams dietary fiber.

Pork and Vegetables with Mustard-Lemon Sauce

Pork is the ideal slow cooker companion for winter squash: the squash adds bright color and understated sweetness to the meal. Look for a beautiful assortment of squash (also called gourds) including acorn, butternut, Hubbard, or turban during fall and winter. Squash is an outstanding source of beta carotene, vitamins A and C, and potassium.

Ingredients:

1 (3 to 4-pound) boneless pork shoulder roast

1 pound carrots, peeled, cut to 2-inch pieces

4 large shallots, peeled, quartered

2 cups peeled butternut squash, cubed

6 to 8 cloves garlic, peeled, cut in half

1 cup apple juice or apple cider

1 tablespoon apple cider vinegar

1 tablespoon grainy mustard

2 teaspoons chicken bouillon granules

1 lemon, zest removed, juiced

¼ cup cold water blended with 1 tablespoon cornstarch

> ***Toast squash seeds:*** after scooping seeds from squash rinse under cold running water; dry. Place on rimmed baking sheet spritz lightly with cooking spray and season with salt, pepper, and/or seasoning blend; and toast in 350°F oven for 8 to 10 minutes until crisp.

Directions: Trim fat from pork roast; if necessary cut roast to fit in slow cooker; season with salt and pepper. Layer carrots, shallots, butternut squash, and garlic cloves in 4-quart slow cooker; place roast on top of vegetables. In a small bowl whisk together apple juice, apple cider vinegar, mustard, chicken bouillon granules, lemon zest and lemon juice; add to slow cooker. Cover and cook on low for 9 to 10 hours or on high for 5 to 6 hours. Do not disturb during cooking and avoid removing cover. When time is up remove pork and vegetables to serving platter; cover to keep warm. Strain cooking liquid into medium saucepot set over medium high heat. Bring liquid to boil; whisk in cornstarch water and continue boiling until liquid thickens to gravy, season as needed. Carve roast and serve with vegetables and sauce. Garnish with toasted squash seeds.

Nutrition: Serves 8. Each serving provides 337 calories, 34 grams protein, 10 grams fat, 25 grams carbohydrate, 5 grams dietary fiber.

End Pages

The following WLS Four Rules and Basic Tenets are widely accepted by bariatric surgeons and nutritionists as lifestyle guidelines to be followed by people who have undergone all manner of gastric surgery for weight loss. I have found that making these tenets a lifestyle is the most effective way for me and many others to manage weight loss and maintain it with weight loss surgery. Refer to the documentation provided you at the time of your surgery for the specifics advised by your bariatric center

Four Rules: Weight Loss Surgery basics

As patients we are well aware that WLS is frequently perceived by outsiders as an easy means to weight loss that requires little or no effort by the patient. It turns out there is nothing easy about the post-WLS lifestyle. At the time of surgery we agreed to follow Four Rules of dietary and lifestyle management guidelines for the rest of our life in order to lose weight and maintain a healthy weight. This is our burden and our responsibility if we wish to keep morbid obesity in remission.

All surgical weight loss procedures including gastric bypass, adjustable gastric banding (lap-band) and gastric sleeve, promote weight loss by decreasing energy (caloric) intake with a reduced or restricted stomach size. The small stomach pouch is only effective when a patient rigorously follows the Four Rules: eat a high protein diet; drink lots of water; avoid snacking on empty calorie food; engage in daily exercise.

In our introduction to a bariatric program we were taught *and agreed* to follow the standard Four Rules which work in concert with our surgically altered stomach and digestive system to bring about rapid massive weight loss. In fact, most of us were asked during the psychological evaluation if we could commit to following the Four Rules. Like me, I bet you said "Of course" with complete confidence. What I missed in the orientation was that these rules would be a way of life for the *rest* of my life. The Four Rules and other WLS dietary basics are discussed in greater detail in Chapter 9. For now let's take a quick look at each rule as it applies to WLS patients.

Protein First: At every meal the WLS patient will eat lean animal, dairy, or vegetable protein before any other food. Protein shakes or supplements may be included as part of the weight loss surgery diet. Patients are advised to consume 60-105 grams of protein a day. Eating lean protein will create a tight feeling in the surgical stomach pouch: this feeling is the signal to stop eating. Many patients report discomfort when eating lean protein, yet this discomfort is the very reason the stomach pouch is effective in reducing food and caloric intake. Animal products are the most nutrient rich source of protein and include fish, shellfish, poultry, and meat. Dairy protein, including eggs, yogurt, and cheese, is another excellent source of protein.

Lots of Water: Like most weight loss programs, bariatric surgery patients are instructed to drink lots of water throughout the day. Most centers advise a minimum of 64 fluid ounces of water each day. Water hydrates the organs and cells and facilitates the metabolic processes of human life. Water flushes toxins and waste from the body. Patients are strongly discouraged from drinking carbonated beverages. In addition, patients are warned against excessive alcohol intake as it tends to have a quicker and more profound intoxicating affect compared with pre-surgery consumption. In addition, non-nutritional beverages of any kind may lead to weight gain and increased snacking.

No Snacking: Patients are discouraged from snacking which may impede weight loss and lead to weight gain. Specifically, patients are forbidden to partake of traditional processed carbohydrate snacks, such as chips, crackers, baked goods, and sweets. Patients who return to snacking on empty calorie non-nutritional food defeat the restrictive nature of the surgery and weight gain results. It is seemingly contradictory that the 5DPT allows snacking. High protein snacks are allowed because they keep the metabolism active, they satiate hunger, and they help relieve the symptoms of carbohydrate withdrawal.

Daily Exercise: In general patients are advised to engage in 30 minutes of physical activity on most days of the week. The most effective way to heal the body from the ravages of obesity is to exercise. Exercise means moving the body: walking, stretching, bending, inhaling and exhaling. Exercise is the most effective, most enjoyable, most beneficial gift one can receive when recovering from life threatening, crippling morbid obesity. Consistent exercise will keep morbid obesity in remission and help compensate for lapses in following the three other rules. People who successfully maintain their weight exercise daily.

Slider Foods & Liquid Restrictions

Slider Foods: To the weight loss surgery patient slider foods are the bane of good intentions often causing dumping syndrome, weight loss plateaus, and eventually weight gain. By definition slider foods are soft simple processed carbohydrates of little or no nutritional value that slide right through the surgical stomach pouch without providing nutrition or satiation. The most commonly consumed slider foods include pretzels, crackers (saltines, graham, Ritz®, etc.) filled cracker snacks such as Ritz Bits®, popcorn, cheese snacks (Cheetos®) or cheese crackers, tortilla chips with salsa, potato chips, sugar-free cookies, cakes, and candy.

The very nature of the surgical gastric pouch is to cause feelings of tightness or restriction when one has eaten enough food. However, when soft simple carbohydrates are eaten this tightness or restriction does not result and one can continue to eat, unmeasured amounts of food without ever feeling uncomfortable. Many patients unknowingly turn to slider foods for this very reason. They do not like the discomfort that results when the pouch is full from eating a measured portion of lean animal or dairy protein, and it is more comfortable to eat the soft slider foods. Slider foods have played a significant role in every case of post-WLS weight regain that I have ever heard about.

Liquid restrictions: After surgical weight loss patients are advised to avoid drinking liquids 30 minutes before meals and 30 minutes after meals. *(The time restriction varies from surgeon to surgeon, but most use the 30 minutes before, 30 minutes after restriction. Follow your surgeon's specific directions.)* In addition there should be no liquid consumed while eating. Following these liquid restrictions allows the pouch to feel tight sooner and stay tight longer, thus leaving the patient feeling satiated for greater periods of time without experiencing the urge to snack. In addition, the longer food stays in the small gastric pouch the more opportunity the body has to absorb nutrients from that food. The liquid restrictions should be followed when eating all meals and snacks, including protein shakes, protein bars, hearty soups, and solid protein main dishes.

Appendix B: 5 Day Pouch Test by Kaye Bailey

The 5 Day Pouch Test (5DPT) is a back-to-basics program that has helped thousands of people around the world take control of the surgical tool and pursue better health with better habits and practices. It is only five days. And during those five days participants learn their pouch is working; they take control of eating and snacking behaviors; and they restore the determination that took them to surgery in the first place..

Days 1 and 2 of the plan are healing days. Participants treat their surgical pouch like a newborn with gentle liquids and soups. Pouch inflammation is reduced and processed carbohydrate cravings subside. Mental focus is on listening to and respecting your body. Days 1 and 2 mimic the early days and weeks following bariatric surgery.

Day 3 introduces soft proteins like canned fish, fresh soft fish or eggs. This is the day we focus on tasting our food, chewing well, and enjoying the goodness of lean-clean protein. We focus on portion control and the liquid restrictions. On this day we start to remember what a tight pouch feels like and we appreciate the feeling of fullness.

Day 4 brings us to firm proteins like ground meat (beef, poultry, lamb, or game) and shellfish, scallops, lobster, salmon or halibut steaks. This is the day we truly realize the power of the pouch and most people are happily surprised to learn their pouch is not broken or stretched back to normal stomach size. The carbohydrate withdrawal is over, and energy levels are improving.

Day 5 finishes the test with solid proteins such as white meat poultry, beef steak, and any of the firm proteins from Day 4. The liquid restrictions are now a habit and we have successfully removed the slider foods from our diet. We have energy for exercise and for the daily tasks of living. Most importantly, we know our weight loss surgery tool works and we now have the confidence and capability to work the tool.

Appendix C: Day 6-Beyond the 5DPT by Kaye Bailey

Day 6 is the way we will eat every day for the rest of our lives. Having successfully broken a carb-cycle, gained a feeling of control over the surgical gastric pouch, and possibly losing a few pounds one is ready for re-entry into a compliant way of eating. This means focusing on protein dense meals, observing the liquid restrictions, and avoiding starches, particularly processed carbohydrates and slider foods. Three meals a day should be two-thirds protein, one-third healthy carbohydrate in the form of low-glycemic vegetables and fruits. Consumption of whole grains is not forbidden, but should be limited to one serving a day.

Appendix D: Food Safety Basics

Provided by United States Department of Agriculture
Food Safety & Inspection Service
http://www.usda.gov

Safe steps in food handling, cooking, and storage are essential to prevent food borne illness. You can't see, smell, or taste harmful bacteria that may cause illness. Most food borne illness may be prevented by following strict food handling, cooking, and storage basics. Be vigilant in your kitchen and protect your health and wellness from food illness.

Shopping: Purchase refrigerated or frozen items after selecting your non-perishables. Never choose meat or poultry in packaging that is torn or leaking. Do not buy food past "Sell-By," "Use-By," or other expiration dates.

Storage and Freshness: Always refrigerate perishable food within 2 hours (1 hour when the temperature is above 90 °F). Check the temperature of your refrigerator and freezer with an appliance thermometer. The refrigerator should be at 40 °F or below and the freezer at 0 °F or below.

Cook or freeze fresh poultry, fish, ground meats, and variety meats within 2 days; other beef, veal, lamb, or pork, within 3 to 5 days. Perishable food such as meat and poultry should be wrapped securely to maintain quality and to prevent meat juices from getting onto other food.

To maintain quality when freezing meat and poultry in its original package, wrap the package again with foil or plastic wrap that is recommended for the freezer.

In general, high-acid canned food such as tomatoes, grapefruit, and pineapple can be stored on the shelf for 12 to 18 months. Low-acid canned food such as meat, poultry, fish, and most vegetables will keep 2 to 5 years — if the can remains in good condition and has been stored in a cool, clean, and dry place. Discard cans that are dented, leaking, bulging, or rusted.

Preparation: Always wash hands with warm water and soap for 20 seconds before and after handling food. Don't cross-contaminate. Keep raw meat, poultry, fish, and their juices away from other food. After cutting raw meats, wash cutting board, utensils, and countertops with hot, soapy water. Cutting boards, utensils, and countertops can be sanitized by using a solution of 1 tablespoon of unscented, liquid chlorine bleach in 1 gallon of water.

Thawing Methods: Refrigerator: The refrigerator allows slow, safe thawing. Make sure thawing meat and poultry juices do not drip onto other food. Cold Water: For faster thawing, place food in a leak-proof plastic bag. Submerge in cold tap water. Change the water every 30 minutes. Cook immediately after thawing. Microwave: Cook meat and poultry immediately after microwave thawing.

> ### *Food Safety Basics*
> Cleanliness: Wash hands & surfaces often.
> Separate: Do not cross-contaminate.
> Heat: Cook to proper temperatures.
> Chill: Refrigerate promptly.

Cooking:
Beef, veal, and lamb steaks, roasts, and chops may be cooked to 145°F.
All cuts of pork, 145°F (New FDA guidelines approved June 2011).
Ground beef, veal and lamb to 160°F.
All poultry should reach a safe minimum internal temperature of 165°F.

Serving: When serving food at a buffet, keep food hot with chafing dishes, slow cookers, and warming trays. Keep food cold by nesting dishes in bowls of ice or use small serving trays and replace them often. Perishable food should not be left out more than 2 hours at room temperature, less if ambient temperature is hot.

Hot food should be held at 140°F or warmer.

Cold food should be held at 40°F or colder.

Leftovers: Discard any food left out at room temperature for more than 2 hours (1 hour if the temperature was above 90°F). Place food into shallow containers and immediately put in the refrigerator or freezer for rapid cooling. Use cooked leftovers within 4 days.

Safe Minimum Cooking Temperatures: Use this chart and a food thermometer to ensure that meat, poultry, seafood, and other cooked foods reach a safe minimum internal temperature. Remember, you can't tell whether meat is safely cooked by looking at it. Any cooked, uncured red meats – including pork – can be pink, even when the meat has reached a safe internal temperature.

Why the Rest Time is Important: After you remove meat from a grill, oven, or other heat source, allow it to rest for the specified amount of time. During the rest time, its temperature remains constant or continues to rise, which destroys harmful germs.

Category	Food	Temperature	Rest Time
Ground Meat & Meat Mixtures	Beef, Pork, Veal, Lamb, Turkey, Chicken	160°F	None
Fresh Beef, Veal, Lamb, game	Steaks, roasts, chops, stew meat	145°F	3 mins.
Poultry	Chicken and turkey whole; poultry breasts, roasts, thighs, legs, wings; duck and goose	165°F	None
Pork and Ham	Fresh pork; fresh ham (raw); pre-cooked ham (reheat temperature)	145°F	3 mins.
Eggs	Eggs	Yolks and whites cooked firm	None
Egg dishes, leftovers, casseroles	Egg dishes such as soufflé or breakfast casseroles: items requiring reheating before serving	160-165°F	None
Seafood	**Fin Fish:** Cook until flesh is opaque and separates easily with a fork. **Shrimp, lobster, crabs:** Cook until flesh is pearly and opaque. **Clams, oysters, and mussels:** Cook until shells open during cooking. **Scallops:** Cook until flesh is milky white or opaque and firm. No resting time needed.		

Provided by FoodSafety.gov U.S. Department of Health & Human Services © 2012

Glossary

Anchovy Paste is an appealing combination of pounded anchovies, vinegar, spices and water comes in tubes and is convenient for many cooking purposes. A small amount adds salty-savory flavor without overpowering a dish. Find anchovy paste by the canned fish in your grocery store or look for it in gourmet specialty shops. Try Beef Puttanesca over Noodles, page 158.

Bariatric Hybrid Tummy a description coined by Kaye Bailey to describe someone who has undergone a bariatric surgical procedure for weight loss including gastric bypass, adjustable gastric banding (lap-band), gastric sleeve, and other. One who has not had a bariatric procedure is described as *organic tummy*.

Basal Metabolic Rate (BMR) is a measure of the energy a body needs to meet its basic needs such as breathing, blood circulation, and cellular growth and repair. This is also known as energy use at rest and generally accounts for one-half to two-thirds of daily energy expenditure.

Body Mass Index (BMI): an index of a person's weight in relation to height; determined by dividing the weight (in kilograms) by the square of the height (in meters).

Buttermilk: commercially available cultured buttermilk is milk that has been pasteurized and homogenized (if 1% or 2% fat), and then inoculated with a culture of lactic acid bacteria to simulate the naturally occurring bacteria in the old-fashioned traditional buttermilk that was the byproduct of butter churned from cream. Buttermilk contains 90.5% water, 3.5% protein, and 1-2% butterfat. Buttermilk is available in dried powder form, similar to powdered milk, shelved in the same location at the market. Powdered buttermilk stores well at room temperature and is usually used in baked goods. A buttermilk dip is essential to crispy oven-fried protein. Try Crispy Oven-Fried Chicken, page 85.

Centers for Disease Control (CDC) is one of the major operating components of the Department of Health and Human Services. It serves as an information gathering agency collaborating government, community and private resources to create the expertise, information, and tools that people and communities need to protect their health with a focus on health promotion, prevention of disease, injury and disability, and preparedness for new health threats.

Cornstarch: a dense, flour-like powder obtained from the endosperm of the corn kernel. Cornstarch is most commonly used as a thickening agent for puddings, sauces, soups, etc. Because it tends to form lumps, cornstarch is generally mixed with a small amount of cold liquid to form a thin paste before being stirred into a hot mixture. Sauces thickened with cornstarch will be clear, rather than opaque, as with flour-based sauces. Try Crispy Oven-Fried Chicken, page 85.

Day 6: a strategy for weight management following completion of the 5 Day Pouch Test. See Appendix C on page 179 for a brief review.

Daily Protein Intake (DPI : the amount of protein, in grams, one should consume in a day. See Protein First: A Really Big Deal on page 19 to learn more.

Edamame are green, immature soybeans rich in antioxidants and vegetable protein. Look for frozen shelled edamame in the freezer case at the market, usually in the organic food section. A 1/2-cup serving provides 9 grams protein, 8 grams carbohydrate and 4 grams dietary fiber. Fresh or frozen edamame are a good source thiamin, iron, magnesium, Vitamin K, folate and manganese.

Exercise (Daily Exercise-Rule #4) See Appendix A: WLS Four Rules on page 176 for a detailed summary.

5 Day Pouch Test (5DPT): See Appendix B on page 178 for a brief overview.

Four Rules of WLS dietary and lifestyle guidelines routinely prescribed by bariatric programs for all weight loss surgery procedures. Rule 1: Protein First; Rule 2: Lots of Water; Rule 3: No Snacking; Rule 4: Daily Exercise. See Appendix A on page 176 for a detailed summary.

Gastric-Blended Household a description coined by Kaye Bailey to describe households in which some members have undergone a bariatric surgical procedure for weight loss *(bariatric hybrid tummy)* while other household members have not *(organic tummy)*.

Gluten (from Latin gluten, "glue") is a protein composite found in foods processed from wheat and related grain species, including barley and rye. It gives elasticity to dough, helping it to rise and to keep its shape, and often gives the final product a chewy texture. Most (but not all) flours contain gluten in varying amounts.

Hoisin Sauce, also called Peking sauce, this thick, reddish-brown sweet and spicy sauce is made from soybeans, garlic, chile peppers, and spices. It is used as a flavoring agent for meat and vegetable stir fry dishes. Bottled hoisin should be refrigerated after opening. Use sparingly; a small amount provides big flavor.

Organic Tummy describes a person who has *not* had a bariatric procedure. The term, coined by Kaye Bailey, is the opposite of bariatric hybrid tummy describing one who has undergone a bariatric surgical procedure for weight loss including gastric bypass, adjustable gastric banding (lap-band), vertical sleeve gastrectomy, and others.

Oyster crackers are small, salted, crackers, typically 1/2-inch rounds or slightly smaller hexagonal shapes. They are popular in the northeastern United States, where they are served as an accompaniment to soup, and in the Cincinnati area, where they are typically served with the city's distinctive chili. Despite their name, oyster crackers do not contain oysters. Try Maryland Oven-Fried Chicken, page 87.

Paillard a French cooking term meaning a 1/3-inch thick slice of meat, usually veal or white meat poultry, pounded very thin and rapidly grilled or pan broiled.

Panko. Japanese bread crumbs used in traditional Japanese cooking for coating fried foods. They're coarser than those normally used in the United States and create a deliciously crunchy crust. Check out the great recipes using panko in the Crispy Crusty Crunchy Coated Protein chapter, page 77.

Pearled barley: a grain commonly used in soups and salads, barley is FDA approved to be labeled as cholesterol lowering proven to reduce the risk of heart disease. Pearled barley is quick cooking and adds a meaty grain to soups and salads. Look for it near the rice and dried beans. Try Grandma's Mushroom Barley Soup, page 64.

Protein Factor: A number used to calculate Daily Protein Intake (DPI). The calculation: Weight (kg) x Protein Factor = Grams DPI. The Protein Factor is selected based on age, level of activity, or current condition. Learn more in Chapter 1: Protein First: A Really Big Deal! on page 19.

Protein First (Rule #1) See Appendix A on page 176 for a detailed summary.

Recommended Dietary Allowance (RDA): the average daily amount of a nutrient considered adequate to meet the known nutrient needs of practically all healthy people. May be used to set nutritional goals for dietary intake by individuals. RDI standards are set by the Institute of Medicine of the National Academies.

Slider Foods See Appendix A on page 176 for a detailed summary.

Snacking (No Snacking – Rule #3) See Appendix A on page 176 for a detailed summary.

Soba noodles. Japanese pasta made from buckwheat flour. Buckwheat is milled from a fruit seed, so it is not a true grain. Soba noodles are complex carbohydrates with high protein content. Studies suggest including soba noodles as part of a healthy diet may lower blood glucose levels. Look for soba noodles on the Asian food aisle of your local market. Try Chicken and Soba Noodle Soup, page 68.

Thermic effect of food is the energy the body uses to digest, absorb, transport and store food. Digesting food accounts for about 10 percent of the body's energy burn. Of the three nutrients (protein, fat, carbohydrates) protein requires the most energy to burn; it has the highest thermic effect.

Vinaigrette: a basic oil-and-vinegar emulsion typically used to dress salad greens, vegetables, and sauce or marinate meat or fish. The basic formula is 3 parts oil to 1 part vinegar which are blended, whisked, or shaken to create an emulsified dressing (upon standing the emulsion will separate.) Vinaigrettes are seasoned with salt, pepper, herbs, garlic, onions, mustard or other flavorful tertiary ingredients. Take a look at the 2B/1B Salads chapter for vinaigrette recipes, beginning on page 27.

Water (Lots of Water – Rule #2) See Appendix A on page 176 for a detailed summary.

Notes:

Bibliography

Abrams, D.; Immediato, L. (2002). *The Best of Gourmet Featuring the Flavors of San Francisco.* New York: Random House, Inc.

Anne Rohaiem, E. E. (2011). *Prevention Best Weight Loss Recipes.* New York: Rodale Inc.

Barham K. Abu Dayyeh, M. D. (2011, March). Gastrojejunal Stoma Diameter Predicts Weight Regain after Roux-en-Y Gastric Bypass. *Clinical Gastroenterology and Hepatology*, 228-233.

Beranbaum, R. L. (1988). *The Cake Bible.* New York: William Morrow and Company, Inc.

Blessing, M. (2004). *Red, White & Blue Ribbon 2004.* Denver: 3D Press, Inc.

Cain, A. C. (2001). *Cooking Light 5-Ingredient 15-Minute Cookbook.* Birmingham: Oxmoor House, Inc.

Cain, A. C. (2003). *Cooking Light Superfast Suppers.* Birmingham: Oxmoor House, Inc.

California Department of Public Health. (2010). *Recommendations to Consumers REgarding Washing Ready-To-Eat Lettuce/Leafy Green Salads.* Sacramento: The State of California, USA.

Culpepper, M. K. (2009). *Cooking Light The Essential Dinner Tonight Cookbook.* Birmingham: Oxmoor House, Inc.

Famularo, J. (1998). *Good & Garlicky Thick & Hearty Soul-Satisfying More-Than-Minestrone Italian Soup Cookbook.* New York: Workman Publishing Company, Inc.

Guasti, C. A. (1998). *Eat Well, Stay Well: 500 Delicious Recipes Made with Healing Foods.* Pleasantville, NY: Reader's Digest Association, Inc.

Howard J. Eisenson, M. a. (2007). *The Duke Diet: The World-Renowned Program for Healthy and Lasting Weight Loss.* New York: Ballantine Books.

Institute of Medicine. (2010). *Strategies to Reduce Sodium Intake in the United States.* College Park, MD: FDA.

Ioannis Raftopoulos; et al. (2011, November). Protein intake compliance of morbidly obese patients undergoing bariatric surgery and its effect on weight loss and biochemical parameter. *Surgery for Obesity and Related Diseases, 7*(6), 733-742.

Jeffrey I. Mechanick, M. F. (2008, April). Medical guidelines for clinical practice for the perioperative nutritional, metabolic, and nonsurgical support of the bariatric surgery patient. *Endocrine Practice*, 318-336.

Judith J. Wurtman, P., & Nina Frusztajer Marquis, M. (2006). *The Serotonin Power Diet.* New York City: Rodale.

Kafka, B. (1995). *Roasting: A Simple Art.* New York: William Morrow and Company, Inc.

Kafka, B. (1998). *Soup A Way of Life.* New York: Artisan.

Kamman, M. (1997). *The New Making of a Cook.* New York: William Morrow and Company, INC.

Keitt, D. (2001). *Gourmet's Casual Entertaining.* New York: Random House for Conde Nast Books.

Knox, G. M. (1987). *New Crockery Cooker Cook Book.* Des Moines: Meredith Corporation.

Laning, T. (2004). *15 Minutes or Less Low-Carb Recipes.* Des Moines: Meredith Corporation.

Lois L. Tlusty. (1986). *Betty Crocker's Cookbook New and Revised.* Racine: Western Publishing Company, Inc.

Louis Weber. (2008). *Crock-Pot The Original Slow Cooker Recipe Collection.* Lincolnwood: Publications International.

Michael R. Eades, M. e. (1996). *Protein Power.* New York: Random House: Bantam Books.

Mildred Ying. (1986). *The New Good Housekeeping Cookbook.* New York: Hearst Books.

Petersen, K. B. (2012). *365 Days of Slow-Cooking.* American Fork, UT: Covenant Communications, Inc.

Rohaiem, A. (2011). *Prevention Best Weight Loss Recipes.* New York: Rodale.

Scarbrough, W. (2011). *Cooking Light The Complete Quick Cook.* New York: Oxmoor House, Inc.

Silvia Leite Faria, Et.Al. (2011). Dietary Protein Intake and Bariatric Surgery Patients: A Review. *Obesity Surgery, Volume: 21*(Issue: 11), 1798-1805.

Smith, A. (2001). *Back to the Table: The Reunion of Food and Family.* New York: Hyperion.

Stephanie. (2009, January). *5 Day Pouch Test Bulletin.*

Suzanne Havala, M. R. (2001). *Being Vegetarian for Dummies.* Hoboken: Wiley Publishing, Inc.

Swilley, D. R. (2008, March). Micronutrient and Macronutrient Needs in Roux-en-Y Gastric Bypass Patients. *Bariatric Times.*

Vollstedt, M. (2000). *The Big Book of Casseroles.* San Francisco: Chronicle Books.

Weldon Owen Inc. (2004). *The New Mayo Clinic Cookbook.* San Francisco: Oxmoor House.

Wesler, C. A. (2000). *The Complete Cooking Light Cookbook.* Birmingham: Oxmoor House, Inc.

Whitney, E., & Rolfes, S. R. (2005). *Understanding Nutrition: Tenth Edition.* Belmont, CA: Thomas Learning, Inc.

Wittgrove, A. C. (1999). *Discharge Instructions for Gastric Bypass.* San Diego: Alvarado Center for Surgical Weight Control.

Wyatt, Nancy Fitzpatrick. (2005). *Cooking Light Annual Recipes 2006.* Birmingham: Oxmoor House, Inc.

Wyatt, Nancy Fitzpatrick. (2006). *Cooking Light Annual Recipes 2007.* Birmingham: Oxmoor House, Inc.

Connections: We are all in this together.

Our human evolution shows that our social connections are as essential to life as are food and water. We need one another to lean upon and to learn from and to lend support. Every human culture on Earth has a social structure through which the group connects for its very survival. In this age of electronic social media we are forming new social structures where people are brought together by similar experiences, beliefs, and goals. Through the Internet weight loss surgery patients from around the world have connected in the now-shuttered LivingAfterWLS Neighborhood, on the major social media sites, and other WLS-specific online communities. We never have to travel this path alone without the benefit and knowledge of others who understand. So let's connect. We are all in this together!

Facebook
http://www.facebook.com/LivingAfterWLS
Pinterest
http://pinterest.com/kayebaileylawls/
YouTube
http://www.youtube.com/user/KayeBailey
Google+
https://plus.google.com - Search Kaye Bailey
Twitter
https://twitter.com/LivingAfterWLS
Email:
KayeBailey@LivingAfterWLS.com

Index

191

Parmesan-Crusted Baked Cod	105
Pecan Crusted Baked Salmon	106
Pecan-Crusted Trout	107
Pineapple Glazed White Fish, Broccoli	137
Skillet Salmon with Mushroom Sauce	136
Tuna and White Bean Salad	46
Wilted Spinach and Tilapia Salad	48

Grains

Beef vegetable Soup with Barley	65
Chicken and Barley Soup	66
Grandma's Mushroom Barley Soup	64

Pork

Autumnal Pork Roast Meal	173
BLT Salad with Toasted Pecans	45
Chili Lime Pork with Sweet Potatoes	148
Chipotle Meatballs and Veggie Soup	72
Garlic-Pepper Pork Chops, Peach Glaze	135
Green Chili with Pork Tenderloin	74
Hot and Sour Pork Soup	73
Italian Sausage Soup	70
Old Dutch Pork with Cabbage	155
Orchard Fresh Ham and Turkey Salad	39
Parmesan-Sage Crusted Pork Chops	99
Pork Chops w/Lemon-Mustard Sauce	132
Pork Chops with Onions and Apples	133
Pork Medallions Creamy Apple Sauce	134
Pork and Vegetables with Sauce	174
Smothered Pork Chops	172
Top-Crusted Pork Loin Chops	100

Shellfish

Black Bean and Shrimp Salsa Salad	47
Crab and Grapefruit Salad	49
Scallop and Fresh Greens Salad	50
Shrimp Fra Diavolo	138

Shrimp Caesar Salad	39
Skillet-Fried Coconut Shrimp	109

Turkey

Black Bean Turkey Tacos	126
California Turkey Avocado Salad	39
Moist Tender Traditional Turkey	146
Smoked Turkey and Melon Salad	41
Sweet Italian Turkey Sausage, Veggies	125
Turkey Chili	75
Turkey and Egg Chilled Lunch Plate	146
Turkey Filled Colorful Peppers	171
Turkey Salad with Oranges	44
Turkey Scaloppini with Romaine Salad	124
Turkey Tenderloin with Mushrooms	123
Turkey Tenderloin Paprikash	169

Vegetables

Autumn Vegetable Minestrone	63
Beef and Broccoli Stir-Fry	128
Beef Vegetable Soup with Barley	65
Chipotle Meatballs and Veggie Soup	72
Grandma's Mushroom Barley Soup	64
Marinara Sauce	92
Mashed Garlic Cauliflower	127
Old Dutch Pork with Cabbage	155
Orchard Fresh Ham and Turkey Salad	39
Pineapple Glazed White Fish, Broccoli	137
Provence-Style Baked Beef, Vegetables	154
Quick Cajun Coleslaw	103
Roasted Brussels Sprouts with Pecans	98
Steamed Spaghetti Squash	138
Sun-Dried Tomato Soup	61
Sweet Italian Turkey Sausage, Veggies	125
Tomato and Cheese Tortellini Soup	62
Turkey Filled Colorful Peppers	171

About Kaye Bailey

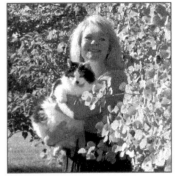

Kaye Bailey developed the 5 Day Pouch Test in 2007 and is the owner of LivingAfterWLS and the 5 Day Pouch Test websites. Ms. Bailey, a professional research journalist and bariatric RNY (gastric bypass) patient since 1999, brings professional research methodology and personal experience to her publications focused on long-lasting successful weight management after surgery.

Concerned about weight regain her bariatric surgeon advised her to "get back to basics". With that vague advice, Ms. Bailey says, "I read thousands of pages and conducted interviews with medical professionals including surgeons, nutritionists, and mental health providers. I collected data from WLS post-ops who honestly and generously shared their experience. My research background gave me the methodology to collect a vast amount of data. As a patient, I found answers to the questions and concerns I have in common with most patients after WLS."

Kaye Bailey is the author of countless articles syndicated in several languages, and books available in print and electronic format including The 5 Day Pouch Test Owner's Manual 2nd Edition 2012, (1st Edition 2008 out-of-print, 50K copies in circulation); Day 6: Beyond the 5 Day Pouch Test (2009 – 3rd Printing January 2015); Cooking with Kaye Methods to Meals: Protein First Recipes You Will Love (2012); and the popular series LivingAfterWLS Shorts.

LivingAfterWLS is proud to produce several free email newsletters each month in support of our ongoing effort to promote healthy weight management with weight loss surgery. Snap on the tag at left to subscribe or visit our websites and click "Newsletters". Each month you can look forward to a new issue of Cooking with Kaye and the 5 Day Pouch Test Bulletin. Enjoy weekly updates in our LivingAfterWLS Weekly Digest. Subscribe now. We value and respect your online information: click the "Privacy" link on any of our web pages to learn more.

The LivingAfterWLS Shorts Series by Kaye Bailey

Vol. 1: 5 Day Pouch Test Express Study Guide

Vol. 2: 5 Day Pouch Test Complete Recipe Collection

Vol. 3: Protein First. Understanding and Living the First Rule of WLS

Vol. 4: Breakfast Basics of WLS

Vol. 5: The Four Rules of Weight Loss Surgery

LivingAfterWLS print Publications by Kaye Bailey are available from Amazon.com, CreateSpace.com and other retail outlets.

LivingAfterWLS eBook Publications by Kaye Bailey are available on Kindle and other devices.

LivingAfterWLS.com   5DayPouchTest.com